Understanding Migraine and Other Headaches

Understanding Health and Sickness Series
Miriam Bloom, Ph.D.
General Editor

Understanding Migraine and Other Headaches

Stewart J. Tepper, M.D.

University Press of Mississippi
Jackson

www.upress.state.ms.us

The University Press of Mississippi is a member of the Association of
American University Presses.

Illustrations by Alan Estridge

11 10 09 08 07 06 05 04 03   4 3 2 1
∞
Library of Congress Cataloging-in-Publication Data
Tepper, Stewart J.
  Understanding migraine and other headaches / Stewart J. Tepper.
    p. cm.
Includes bibliographical references and index.
    ISBN 1-57806-591-7 (cloth : alk. paper) — ISBN 1-57806-592-5
(pbk. : alk. paper)
1. Migraine. 2. Headache. I. Title.
RC392 .T39 2004
616.8′4912—dc22   2003017451

British Library Cataloging-in-Publication Data available

Contents

Introduction

Headaches have bedeviled humanity for all of recorded time. Even in ancient Egypt, suggestions were included in hieroglyphics on how to eliminate severe headache. The Egyptians recommended strapping a crocodile to the top of the head, which might have distracted the sufferer significantly, but advances have brought treatment to a designed, specific level undreamed of even 25 years ago.

Migraine, in particular, is becoming easier to identify and treat. Eighteen percent of women, six percent of men, and four percent of children have migraine. All races are affected, although for reasons that are unknown, whites are affected more than African Americans, and Asian Americans are least often afflicted.

Migraine is an inherited condition; many families can trace it back generations. It can be discouraging for migraine sufferers to see the disease reproduce itself in their children, and realize that the suffering will be perpetuated.

The disease has enormous economic and social consequences, both to individual sufferers and to society as a whole. A large public health study conducted by professors Richard Lipton and Walter Stewart of Albert Einstein and Johns Hopkins Schools of Medicine found that migraine is found more often in people at lower socioeconomic levels. This has been attributed to a downward spiral caused by recurrent disabling headaches. And the cost to U.S. society alone is in excess of $13 billion per year in lost work. This is a not insignificant problem—not "just a headache"—and calls for better education and treatment.

Many productive people have struggled with migraine. It is speculated that Charles Darwin suffered from migraine among other health-related problems that plagued him most of his adult life. Lewis Carroll had migraine with aura, and his visual aura symptoms are felt to be the basis for some of the hallucinatory scenes of *Alice in Wonderland*. Boswell described Samuel Johnson's headaches, which sound very migrainous. Sports figures such as Kareem Abdul-Jabbar in basketball and Terrell Davis in football have fought off migraines during crucial games.

The news from the fight against migraine is good: our understanding of the disease, its causes and its treatment is making huge strides. A revolution in medications for migraine has occurred as a result of improved diagnosis and markedly more sophisticated pharmacology.

This book goes through the story of migraine and other headaches—from their genetics and mechanisms to options for treatments. It is not meant to substitute for a physician, who will provide a patient suffering from headache with diagnosis and, if appropriate, medication. The goal is understanding and knowledge that may be liberating when confronting headache in yourself or in friends, associates, or relatives.

I begin by explaining the types of headaches, and trace the earliest part of a migraine attack to its smoldering conclusion. Then I consider who gets migraine and the possible causes, including remarkable new work in genetics and brain function. Establishing how bad migraines are can lead to more reasonable treatment, and a section on disability will provide a shortcut to obtaining the right treatment, the first time.

Next I explore the medications available and forthcoming, from the most sophisticated designer drugs to the simplest mineral and vitamin supplements.

The chapter on chronic daily headache and other rarer headaches such as cluster or those headaches associated with sex or exercise, suggests that some of these less often seen headaches are often treatable. *Understanding Migraine and Other Headaches* concludes with a discussion of ongoing and potential research, and provides resources for information and help. Overall, I hope that this book will serve as a guide not only for understanding headaches, but also for action.

Understanding Migraine and Other
Headaches

1. What Is Migraine?

The diagnosis of migraine was simplified and standardized when the International Headache Society (IHS) put together diagnostic criteria that are now used worldwide. Revisions in classification will soon be available. The IHS divided headache into two major types, primary and secondary.

Secondary headaches are caused by underlying medical conditions. Immune diseases (such as lupus erythematosis and rheumatoid arthritis), infections (such as meningitis and HIV), metabolic conditions (such as low thyroid function), neurologic conditions (such as high spinal fluid pressure and hemorrhage in the brain), and head trauma can all cause headache. Primary headaches are their own disorder, caused by changes in brain chemistry or recognized brain diseases.

Primary headaches do not harm the body, so they are often referred to as "benign." The three main types of primary headache are migraine, tension-type headache, and cluster. I will first discuss migraine headache and its treatment. Later sections of the book will cover other types of headache.

The IHS has created a checklist by which migraine can be diagnosed. The following criteria define migraine without aura, which used to be called common migraine:

1. The patient should have had at least five of these headaches.
2. The headache lasts from 4 to 72 hours.
3. The headache must have at least two of the following:
   a. One-sided location
   b. Pulsing or throbbing quality
   c. Moderate or severe intensity, inhibiting or prohibiting daily activities

    d. Headache is worsened by routine physical activity, such as bending over or climbing stairs

4. The headache must be accompanied by at least one of the following:

    a. Nausea and/or vomiting

    b. Dislike of light (photophobia) and dislike of noise (phonophobia)

5. Secondary causes of headache are excluded with a normal exam and/or normal CAT scan or MRI scan.

It can be very useful to examine these criteria and take them apart a bit. For example, when a person has a severe, three-day, one-sided headache, and is vomiting and bedridden in a dark, quiet room, it is not difficult to make a diagnosis of migraine.

Where the diagnosis is missed is with moderate migraine. Take a case of a woman with her usual six-hour menstrual headache. The headache is moderate in intensity, steady and not throbbing in quality, and located at the back of her head and in her neck. She is not nauseated.

On the way into work, she puts on sunglasses and turns off the radio, the sound of which is annoying her. When she gets to work, she's not quite firing on all cylinders, and estimates that she is working at about 50% effectiveness. Her headache is a bit worse when she bends to pick up a piece of paper.

This woman has migraine. I think that she herself probably would dismiss it as tension headache, because it was moderate in intensity, not one-sided, nauseating or throbbing, and located in her neck. But remember, migraine does not have to be severe, nauseating, or pulsating.

It is worth going down the checklist so that we can see why this is migraine. First, this is her usual headache, so she has had at least five of them.

The headache lasted six hours. Migraine can last from four to 72 hours, so the headache meets the length criterion for a migraine.

Next, the headache was moderate in intensity, inhibited but did not prohibit her activity, and was worse when she bent to pick up a piece of paper. So, the headache met two of the four criteria listed under #3.

Finally, she apparently had photophobia (she wore sunglasses) and phonophobia (she turned off the car radio), so she met one of the two criteria listed under #4 for migraine. As long as her exam was normal, she had migraine.

It is easy to see how the diagnosis could be missed and how this type of headache could be dismissed as a tension or hormonal headache. IHS criteria do not specify location, so neck pain does not mean tension headache; location does not predict diagnosis.

Indeed, doctors can miss the diagnosis as well. In 1999 a population-based survey was done of people with headache in Maryland. Participants were read the IHS criteria for migraine. Those meeting the criteria were asked whether they knew that they had migraine.

Fifty-two percent of the participants in this survey who met IHS criteria had not received the diagnosis of migraine. So the diagnosis is being missed a lot, and it is probably moderate migraine patients who are being missed, or people who assume they have tension headache because of neck pain, or "sinus headache" because of frontal or cheek pain.

A large international study conducted in primary care physician offices in 2002 found that 94% of patients complaining to their doctors of episodic headaches had migraine-type headaches. Most episodic headaches significant enough to be worth complaining about—those with impact—are migraine.

Simplicity and epidemiology suggest that, given how frequent migraines are, if a person has an established pattern (lasting at least six months) of recurrent headaches (greater than four hours but up to several days in length) and associated with some disability, it is likely that it is migraine and not another headache type. Add to that a family history of headaches, a worsening around the time of menses, or other obvious triggers, and the likelihood of migraine goes even higher. In fact, a stable pattern of disabling headaches occurring in discrete episodes is migraine until proven otherwise.

Aura

An aura is a reversible neurologic event that lasts less than an hour and is followed within an hour by the headache. Migraine with aura used to be called classic migraine. Some people still feel it is necessary to have an aura before the headache to make a diagnosis of migraine, but that is not true.

Auras can be remarkable experiences, and any part of the brain can be involved. Usually, auras are visual. Visual auras are called positive visual phenomena, because people actually see things. That is, instead of "things going black" or "a curtain coming down over vision," as often happens in stroke or warning for stroke, patients with migrainous aura usually have active visual disturbance.

Visual auras are variable. The auras usually take the form of dots, a zigzag, or a shimmering crescent that gradually gets bigger until the person with aura can no longer see. The zigzags have been compared to the old fortifications that were on the battlements of castles; these auras are sometimes referred to as fortification spectra. Patients will sometimes develop tunnel vision or "Swiss cheese" vision, with holes in what they see.

A problem for patients is that positive visual phenomena obscure vision just as badly as if the patient had lost the vision to negative blackness. Aura may begin as a shimmering blind spot and gradually spread until all useful vision is blocked. So for some patients the aura is as big a problem as the headache that follows.

Although auras are most often visual, they can be any neurologic symptom. After visual disturbances, the next most common symptom is numbness or tingling of face, arms or legs. When the aura tingling or numbness ascends from arm to face, it is referred to as *cheiro-oral*. Occasionally, people can get weak on one side (hemiplegic) or have trouble with language (aphasic).

As will be discussed later, there is a genetic component to migraine, shown by a tendency to inherit migraine with and/or without aura. One very rare form called familial hemiplegic migraine involves a long aura of paralysis.

Another unusual type of aura is basilar-type migraine, in which multiple symptoms are generated in the brainstem. Aura symptoms include dizziness, double vision, slurred speech, and, more rarely, loss of consciousness.

Only 15–20% of patients with migraine consistently get aura before their headache. The following IHS criteria are used to diagnose migraine with aura:

1. Reversible brain symptoms
2. Gradual development over five minutes
3. Aura duration of less than one hour
4. Headache follows aura in less than one hour

If the aura lasts longer than one hour, the condition is no longer called migraine with typical aura, but is referred to as migraine with prolonged aura.

Sometimes an aura occurs without being followed by a migraine headache. This is called aura without headache, or migraine equivalent. Some people get all three forms of migraine at different times—migraine with aura, migraine without aura, and typical aura without headache.

Description of a Migraine

Prodrome

Many people with migraine have a premonition, called a *prodrome*, that the headache is coming. A prodrome can occur before an aura or before a migraine without aura.

Some prodromes last for several days, while others can last for six to eight hours and build directly into the migraine.

Prodromes are variable. Some people experience general disturbances of body function, such as fatigue, joint aches, hunger or food cravings, insomnia, or restlessness; others have mental status

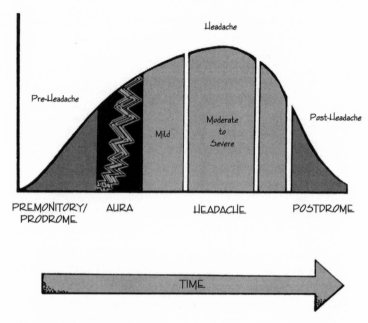

Fig. 1.1 Stages of a Migraine.

changes, such as inattention, lack of concentration, and confusion. A person who experiences dislike of light and noise (photophonophobia), dislike of smells (osmophobia), or nausea during their migraine attacks can experience these symptoms for days before the migraine headache actually begins.

Neck pain can be a prodrome of hours or days, and can then persist into the attacks of pain, confusing patients into thinking they have a tension headache. Finally, some migraine sufferers experience emotional changes such as euphoria or depression during the prodrome.

Not everyone gets a prodrome, but for those who do the symptoms can be quite significant, and can interfere with activities of daily living. It should be stressed that the prodrome can have impact even before the migraine headache hits.

The Migraine Itself

The speed with which the migraine headache comes on is variable. Some people have some nausea or photophonophobia just as the headache begins. Others wake up with a full-blown migraine, sometimes vomiting, sometimes just nauseated.

Those whose headaches develop during the day may not know how fast the headache is going to develop. The headache may build gradually during the day, often with neck pain, with accumulation of nausea and photophonophobia, gradually becoming throbbing. At other times, the whole devastating migraine will be present in 30 minutes, with less chance to intervene medically. The usual course during a day is for the headache and other symptoms to develop over about two to four hours.

In a severe migraine, the headache is often one-sided. Some people have a predominant side on which the headache happens, while others can get it on either side or both sides. Sometimes the headache switches sides; this can happen each day of the migraine. The migraine can be almost anywhere on the head—on the forehead, behind or around the eye, in the cheek or over the sinuses, in the teeth, close to the ear, or in the neck and back of the head. In almost half of patients, the migraine is associated with tearing eye, stuffy nose, running nose, or "post-nasal drip," which leads to an incorrect diagnosis of "sinus headache."

Migraine is generated in the brain, but the location of origin is not where the pain is felt. Migraine appears to be generated from brainstem centers opposite the side of pain, when the pain is one-sided. The anatomy of the nervous system is often crossed and, as with most neurologic diseases, migraine has contralateral activation.

Associated Symptoms of Migraine

Migraine is sometimes diagnosed by the presence of photophonophobia. Many migraine patients have sensitivity to light all the time, not just during a migraine. But during a migraine the sensitivity to light and noise may increase dramatically.

Some people get sensitivity to all stimuli during a migraine. They are sensitive to smells (osmophobia) and to movement and touch, with their other symptoms. This perception of non-painful stimuli as painful is called allodynia.

We now have a picture of a throbbing headache on one or both sides of the head, that gradually or quickly comes on, is associated with nausea, dislike of light and noise, and lasts four hours to three days, but generally about a day. The location of the headache can be in the neck, and the pain can be associated with "sinus-like" symptoms.

Migraine, then, is not just a headache. It is a *syndrome*, which means that it is a collection of symptoms. This collection of symptoms can make a person feel very ill indeed—migraine used to be called the "sick headache." People become disabled, often cannot work for days on end, cannot take care of their families, and can be a burden to others.

Families, fellow workers, and even friends blame patients for having migraine, and often imply that the headaches should be under their control. Even worse, laid low by a brain disease, people with migraine often blame themselves for their incapacity.

Postdrome

Some patients with migraine also have symptoms after the headache, or *postdrome*, to match the prodrome of symptoms before the migraine. Patients describe feeling hung over, somewhat disoriented, sick, or not right for days after the headache subsides. This, too, adds to the disability of an attack, because a person in a migraine postdrome may not be able to function at full capacity for several days after the headache stops.

"Sinus Headache"

Even though the location of the pain is not indicative of the location of the underlying disease process, it is very important to the person getting the migraine. People misinterpret these locations and attribute the cause of the migraine to the fact that they get the headache in that place. Patients who get their headaches over their cheeks or sinuses frequently say they have "sinus headaches." Yet a study completed in 2002 found that, of over 3,000 people with self-diagnosed or doctor-diagnosed "sinus headaches," over 90% met IHS criteria for migraine-type headaches. Less than ten people in the study had sinusitis.

It complicates the picture of migraine that some accompanying symptoms are runny nose, stuffy nose, postnasal drip, or tearing eyes. This is referred to as migraine with vasomotor instability.

It is obvious why people with a migraine and vasomotor instability assume that they have a "sinus headache." But true headache associated with sinusitis is caused by infection and inflammation.

The pain of sinusitis is usually dull and achy, and if there is a bacterial infection, the pain may be accompanied by fever and may last until antibiotics are taken. Migraine occurs for pre-defined periods of time (4–72 hours), while bacterial or viral "sinus headaches" last until they are treated or remit naturally, which does not always happen with a bacterial infection. The medical literature lists headache as a minor, not a major feature of sinusitis.

Further muddying the sinus picture is that when a person gets a severe headache with nausea and photophonophobia, but then gets a runny or stuffy nose, that person often calls the doctor to receive antibiotics. Upon taking prescribed medication, the headache goes away in two or three days, which can be the natural length of a migraine. If the patient had not received the medication, the migraine would have gone away anyway.

So how does one distinguish a migraine from sinusitis-induced headache? First, headaches associated with sinusitis do not generally throb, are not usually associated with photophonophobia, and are not accompanied by nausea.

Second, sinus x-rays of someone with migraine appear generally normal, while sinusitis can cause air fluid separations and other evidence for active infection. True bacterial sinus infections occur less commonly in the general population than do migraines, and viral sinusitis rarely is associated with significant disabling headache.

Migraine patients have a family history of headache. Finally, fever and purulent discharge occur in sinusitis but not in migraine.

A review of the medical literature fails to turn up an entity called "sinus headache." It is likely that this idea was generated by advertising companies marketing sinus medications, rather than by scientific study.

The Neck and Migraine

Those who get neck pain assume that they are having "muscle-contraction headache." The IHS does not recognize this term, as it is not clear that anyone gets headache from contraction of neck muscles. Rather, many specialists believe that at the beginning of migraine, an area of the brainstem turns on like a central generator, and this area in turn activates nerve pathways that go down into the neck, which hurts and often causes muscle tightness.

There are people that develop "neck migraine" from problems in the neck. Certain people have trigger points that seem to respond to injections of medications such as steroids into the soft tissue of the neck.

Other people have abnormalities deeper in the neck, such as in the nerve roots coming out of the upper (cervical) spinal cord. If an anesthesiologist places numbing medication or steroids around one of these and the headache turns off, the patient is said to have "cervicogenic headache."

Without this diagnostic "cervical block," cervicogenic headache can be very hard to distinguish from a migraine located in the neck and back of head. Sometimes a herniated disc (a protrusion of the cartilage that sits between the vertebral bones) irritates the nerve root. Other times, the nerve root is traumatized by an accident. Finally, the nerve can be damaged for no apparent reason.

Because cervicogenic headache is rare and migraine is common, most people who get the severe headache in the back of the neck and head have migraine.

Recently, evidence has mounted that the poison that causes botulism, botulinum neurotoxin, injected in the neck and head, can

prevent migraine. However, it is not clear whether botulinum neurotoxin works by preventing muscles from going into spasm, or from
preventing nerve firing in the neck (which exacerbates the attacks),
breaking a cycle between brainstem and the neck.

In conclusion, migraine can be quite variable, from moderate to
severe, with different qualities, locations, and associated symptoms.
It can be preceded by warning symptoms, such as prodrome and/or
aura, or can occur without warning. It is therefore not surprising
that the diagnosis of migraine is frequently missed, by patient and
doctor alike.

2. Who Gets Migraine?

Migraine is a genetic condition. Ask migraine sufferers whether they have any family members with migraine, and at least 50% will answer yes. But ask the first-degree relatives of a migraine sufferer if they have migraine by describing the characteristics of the headache, and there will almost always be a family member with migraine.

Most migraine is not caused by a single gene. With the rare exception of familial hemiplegic migraine, migraine (with or without aura) is likely to be "polygenic," with multiple genes involved.

Migraine can encompass a spectrum from mild to moderate headache that interferes with activities, to disabling headache accompanied by vomiting and lying in bed for three days, affecting life drastically. And since the diagnosis of migraine is often missed, and instead the headaches are misdiagnosed as tension-type, sinus, or muscle-contraction, when patients are asked about relatives with migraine they frequently respond that they have no relatives with migraine, and certainly not their kind of headaches. It may be better to ask if anyone in the family has any headache at all, or "headacheiness," and then delve in a little more when the answer is yes, which it usually will be.

When patients cannot find that ancestors had headache, they often fail to think about their own children as part of a family history. If a spouse does not have headache, and the child of a migraine patient does, then the likelihood is that the migraine was transmitted genetically from patient to child.

Co-morbidity

Patients with migraine often have other medical or psychiatric conditions. This is referred to as co-morbidity, and the related conditions co-morbid conditions.

For example, depression and anxiety are much more common in migraine patients than people without migraine. Yet these psychiatric conditions do not cause migraine, and migraine does not result in primary depression or anxiety. Co-morbidity implies co-occurrence, not one condition causing the other. Sometimes, depression and anxiety will occur secondary to migraines. It is not clear, however, whether patients inherit a tendency to these psychiatric illnesses when they inherit the migraines.

People with migraine are twice as likely to get depression in their lifetime as people without migraine. And people with depression are twice as likely to get migraine over a lifetime as people without depression.

Epilepsy, too, is co-morbid in migraine patients. One hypothesis is that there is an underlying, inherited neurologic abnormality—a *hyperexcitability*—of the brain, that predisposes people to get these diseases together.

Recurring migraine headaches can occur after an injury to the head or neck, such as a car accident, or follow an infection such as meningitis. We do not know if people who develop migraine in these situations would have developed it anyway due to a genetic tendency, or whether migraine can develop spontaneously.

Gender

During childhood, boys and girls develop migraine with the same frequency. However, with puberty, women begin to develop migraine far more frequently than men. It is during adulthood that a three-to-one prevalence of women to men with migraine is seen.

Up to one quarter of people who will develop migraine do so during the first decade of life. In each of the next four decades, another 20–25% of people develop their first migraine. Less than 5% of patients develop migraine after age 50.

Since 18% of women and only 6% of men have migraine, and the presentation is usually after puberty, migraine is most frequently a disease of adult women. Why this sex difference occurs is unknown, and since migraine occurs in men, it is not purely associated with female hormones and their fluctuation.

Race

Studies from around the world indicate that migraine frequency is lower in Africa and Asia. Further insight into racial prevalence was found in a study published in 1996 by Dr. William Stewart and Dr. Richard Lipton, who reviewed the prevalence of migraine in over 12,000 people in Baltimore County, Maryland. Migraine prevalence was 20% in white women (9% in white men), 16% in African American women (7% in African American men), and 9% in Asian American women (4% in Asian American men). Thus, the racial differences in migraine frequency appear to be genetic.

Socioeconomic Class

An interesting discovery of the past decade was the finding, also by Lipton and Stewart, that migraine in the U.S. is more common in people of lower socioeconomic class. That is, someone with migraine is less likely to have a college education or a high-paying job.

Doctors Lipton and Stewart speculated that the reason for this was a "downward spiral" caused by the recurring migraines themselves. Someone who has disabling headache over and over and misses class time, cannot do homework, or has difficulty keeping a job can experience a downward trend in what he or she can accomplish.

If this speculation is true, correct diagnosis and treatment of migraine is important both to the individual with migraine and to society as a whole. It has been estimated in one study that migraine costs the U.S. $10 billion per year in lost labor.

The reverse trend is seen with episodic tension-type headache; for reasons that are unclear, these patients are more likely to have a college education and higher socioeconomic class. People with chronic tension-type headache and chronic migraine are intermediate in their level of accomplishment and salary.

3. The Role of Hormones

Menstruation

In women, migraines frequently occur at or around ovulation and menstruation. Most women lose their headaches during pregnancies, and often lose them after menopause. Some women have the reverse—worse headaches during pregnancies and after menopause—but they are the exception.

The onset of a migraine around menstruation appears to be triggered by the drop in estrogen during the second half of the cycle as a woman approaches her period. High-dose estrogen, taken just before the day of flow, can blunt or prevent menstrual migraines. Low-dose estrogen, administered by skin patch or pill, is usually ineffective. Pre-treating with estrogen has a chance to work only if the headaches occur at a regular time in relation to the first day of flow. If the cycle is irregular, this approach is not likely to work.

Other medications helpful in preventing menstrual migraine when taken just before a period include the non-steroidal anti-inflammatory drugs, and certain triptans and ergots (see chapter 6).

Birth Control Pills

In the gynecologic journals, many articles suggest that birth control pills can help prevent migraine, while in the neurologic journals many articles suggest that they can worsen migraine and that lower-dose estrogen birth control pills are more likely to be tolerated by women with migraine.

All migraine patients have a slight increase in the risk for stroke compared to people who do not have migraine, although the mechanism for this risk is unknown. Women with migraine with aura have at least a doubled risk for stroke compared to the general population, and a higher risk than women with migraine without aura. The risk of stroke remains very low in menstruating women, about one-tenth as likely as during pregnancy.

Estrogen birth control pills double and may even triple the risk for stroke; if other risk factors for stroke are added, the risk is even higher. It is not known how the factors for vascular risk interact—it is analogous to accumulating risk for heart disease. For example, smoking increases the risk for stroke from three to five times, so smoking and taking birth control pills together raises the risk of stroke significantly. Other risk factors include obesity, high blood pressure, diabetes, and a family history of premature heart disease or stroke.

In migraine with aura, with its increased stroke risk, many headache specialists consider the risk too high to recommend estrogen hormone birth control pills. However, the risk is lower than that for a conventional pregnancy, so the recommendation is controversial. Some specialists allow estrogen birth control pills in women with migraine without aura, but not in women with migraine with aura. Other specialists restrict oral contraceptives only for prolonged aura, or for aura with specific neurologic features, such as hemiparesis.

If I take care of a woman with migraine with aura who is determined to take birth control pills if at all possible, I make a number of recommendations. First, it is worth trying progesterone as a hormone contraceptive. Progesterone-only pills can be given (the "mini-pill"), although they often have an unacceptable risk of bleeding. And progesterone injections (Depo-provera) can be tolerated—although some women get headaches from these shots and are burdened for three months with the effects of the progesterone injection.

Second, it is worth checking for "hidden" risks for stroke that add to the risk for a woman taking estrogen birth control pills: circulating antibodies (referred to as anticardiolipin antibodies) that increase clotting, and certain proteins (proteins C and S) that mediate part of coagulation in the blood, deficiencies of which also increase the risk of thrombosis and stroke. Simple blood tests can establish the presence or absence of these conditions; if they are present, I strongly recommend against taking estrogen birth control pills. I also often recommend a baby aspirin per day, as its anti-platelet effect may decrease the stroke risk. But as noted, since the stroke risk is significantly less than the risk accompanying a pregnancy, I abide by informed patient preference.

Pregnancy

During pregnancy, migraines usually improve as the pregnancy proceeds. If they do not improve or worsen, non-drug therapy is most appropriate, such as keeping regular habits, doing regular aerobic exercise, relaxation exercises, and biofeedback. If medications are needed, simple drugs such as acetaminophen or mild opioid narcotics can be used safely, along with a few anti-nausea medications such as metoclopramide (Reglan) and ondansetron (Zofran). The only preventive medication for migraine currently rated by the FDA as Category B ("no evidence of risk in humans") is cyproheptadine (Periactin), an old-fashioned, sedating antihistamine, with serotonin-blocking effects. Some obstetricians will permit use of more conventional prophylactic anti-migraine agents.

Menopause

A worsening of the intensity or an increase in the frequency of migraines can be a first sign of menopause. However, when a natural menopause is completed, two thirds of women show an improvement or a complete elimination of their migraines. For the other third of patients, the results are mixed—either a worsening or persistence of the headaches.

Some women have a change in pattern to their headaches at menopause. In particular, visual auras occur without migraine headache. These are sometimes called "late life migraine accompaniments."

In one large study, surgical menopause (removal of both ovaries) worsened migraine in two-thirds of patients—the reverse of the ratio for natural menopause. It is possible that during natural menopause, chemical receptors in the brain change in response to the gradual ramping down of estrogen, while acute removal of estrogen does not allow for this slow resetting of these receptors.

The effects of hormone replacement therapy (HRT) at menopause are not usually possible to predict, but there is often a form of HRT that will work and not worsen migraines. If HRT is to be administered, it is important to take estrogen daily and not intermittently, because an estrogen drop could precipitate migraine monthly.

Recently, data from a Women's Health Initiative study found that HRT increased vascular risks in women receiving both estrogen and progesterone replacement, although data from estrogen alone are not complete at the time of this writing. Traditional HRT not only did not reduce the risk of stroke and heart disease, it appeared to increase their frequency, along with breast cancer, although it did reduce osteoporosis.

Thus, enthusiasm for HRT has dropped dramatically. If HRT is recommended for symptomatic relief of menopausal symptoms (e.g., hot flashes) or as treatment for osteoporosis, some headache specialists feel that women with migraine do better with synthetic estrogens such as ethinyl estradiol, rather than horse-derived estrogen such as Premarin. However, there are no scientific data on which to base this conjecture. Switching estrogen can often relieve trouble with a given treatment.

The third concern with HRT is the estrogen dose. Most women do well with a traditional, medium dose, but some require very low dose, while some, paradoxically, do better with high-dose estrogen. The only way to tell is to try one dose, and if it seems to worsen migraines, change the dose up or down in a systematic way.

Some women tolerate the estrogen patch but not the pills, which they find trigger too many migraines. Estrogen can also be given by injection, and can be mixed with testosterone (Estratest); each of these approaches can be tried when simpler measures have triggered migraine.

Finally, synthetic estrogen-like compounds tamoxifen (Nolvadex) and raloxifene (Evista) appear to be worth a try if other forms of estrogen have been ruled out. These medications usually do not trigger migraine. How they stack up against traditional HRT in migraine patients is not known; their effects may be different in terms of the risks of traditional estrogen/progesterone treatment.

4. What Causes Migraine?

The Hyperexcitable Brain

If migraine is inherited, what is it that is inherited? One way to think about this is that migraine patients have a brain that is too excitable, a so-called "hyperexcitable brain." For some reason, specific neurons in the brain—or nuclei—discharge too easily, activating pathways that initiate the mechanism of pain and associated symptoms, and resulting in the migraine syndrome. The tendency to fire is what is inherited.

Nitric Oxide

The brain is composed of nerve cells (neurons) that communicate with each other by chemical and electrical signals. Cells can fire individually or en masse. There are many hypotheses about what it is in neurons that makes them hyperexcitable. One possibility is that migraine nerve cells are too sensitive to nitric oxide, a chemical messenger released by some nerve cells to activate certain others.

An interesting piece of evidence in favor of nitric oxide causing migraine is what happens when people are administered nitroglycerin. This medicine is given to patients with chest pain (angina) caused by blockage of the coronary arteries; it also carries nitric oxide into the brain. People without migraine who take nitroglycerin for angina will get a brief, unpleasant headache afterward. People with migraine who take nitroglycerin get the brief headache, but hours later also get migraine. The theory is that nitric oxide is a cell messenger that causes migraine, but this does not explain why the migraine occurs in bursts or what happens when nitric oxide fulfills its usual functions in the body.

Magnesium

Another theory is that some patients with migraine have too little magnesium in the brain. Low magnesium may lead to nerves becoming hyperexcitable. Low magnesium destabilizes nerves by altering the ability to control the influx and efflux of charged ions, resulting in nerve cells firing too easily.

This low magnesium has been found in the nerves of migraine patients with aura, and in patients with migraine around their menstrual periods. Intravenous magnesium terminates some menstrual migraines. Other patients respond to daily magnesium supplements with a decreased number of migraines. Not everyone given magnesium supplementation benefits (and many patients get diarrhea from the magnesium). The lack of uniform clinical success with magnesium supplementation suggests that the causes of hyperexcitability associated with migraine vary.

Energy Metabolism

The basic storage molecule of energy in the body is adenosine triphosphate, or ATP. This molecule is like a rechargeable battery. Each ATP has three phosphates in a chain on the molecule, and energy is stored in the bonds between them.

When one phosphate is pulled off the ATP, it gives off energy, and these aliquots of energy are used to run everything in the body. However, once the ATP loses a phosphate, it becomes adenosine diphosphate, or ADP. A new phosphate has to be put back onto the ADP to make ATP and thus "recharge" the battery.

The neurons in the brains of some migraine patients have been found to have a problem recharging ADP back to ATP, and the lack of adequately phosphorylated ADP destabilizes the nerves so that they fire more easily. The patient's brain nerves therefore have a tendency to fire due to inadequate regeneration of ATP from ADP.

Certain vitamins help make the ADP into ATP. These vitamins serve as "co-enzymes," chemical midwives without which energy metabolism cannot move to completion. A key co-enzyme is vitamin B2, also called riboflavin, which helps propel a chain movement of electrons during energy reactions. Interestingly, one study showed that some migraine patients who take high-dose vitamin B2 (400 mg/day for 3–4 months) can reduce their migraines (see chapter 7).

Calcium Channels and Familial Hemiplegic Migraine

As noted in chapter 1, the section on aura, hemiplegic migraine is associated with temporary paralysis of one side of the body, occurring during the aura and persisting for hours or even days. The genetic basis for some patients with this very rare form of migraine, familial hemiplegic migraine (FHM), has been identified. One gene that causes it has been mapped to chromosome 19, one to chromosome 4, another to chromosome 1. The genes on chromosomes 1 and 19 code for the calcium channel. (There are many gates or channels in neurons that allow ions with positive or negative charge such as sodium, potassium, or calcium into the cells. These gates open and close and allow for establishing a certain amount of positive and negative charge in a particular cell.) The FHM gene controls the structure of one of the channels in nerve cells.

The mutant calcium channel does not open and close properly and cannot regulate the amount of calcium coming into the cell, so calcium influx and efflux regulation goes awry. This in turn leads to neurons firing too easily.

Ion channel abnormalities are referred to as *channelopathies* and can occur in the gates for sodium, potassium, calcium, and other ions. These channelopathies have been linked to a variety of paroxysmal neurologic conditions—nervous system diseases whose clinical manifestations occur in discrete episodes, such as epilepsy and migraine. The underlying nerve cell channels are abnormal all the time, but the discharges occur periodically, possibly due to gradual toxic buildups of charged ions. Channelopathies may underlie the co-morbidity of migraine and epilepsy.

Because abnormal calcium channels are a cause of FHM, blocking them with a calcium channel blocker specifically treats this form of migraine. Other channelopathies may cause other types of migraines.

Problems exist with all theories for the causes of migraine. One is that not all patients with migraine have low magnesium, nor do they all respond to magnesium, vitamin B2, or calcium channel blockers. Another unknown is why any of these problems, which are constant, make nerve cells fire only occasionally—and why, when they do, they often fire only on one side of the brain. Migraine is polygenic. We still have a way to go in understanding what patients inherit that causes migraine, but we are a lot closer than we were a decade ago.

Events in the Brain Leading to Migraine

The Mechanism of Aura

We used to think that aura was caused by blood vessels constricting, and migraine headache caused by blood vessels dilating. In that theory, aura was caused by too little blood to the brain, and throbbing migraine pain by too much. However, it is now known that some blood vessels constrict during the headache, and that some vessels dilate during aura.

In some animals, a process called *cortical spreading depression* has been found. In this phenomenon, abnormal nerves fire in the visual area at the back of the brain; this activation spreads forward across the brain at a rate of three millimeters per minute. In the wake of the activation, the nerves are quiescent for a period of time; this period is referred to as cortical spreading depression (even though it is in reality cortical spreading *activation*). The initial firing is associated with an increase in blood flow, and the spreading depression with decreased blood flow (but not such a low flow that nerve cells are deprived of oxygen).

Is the spreading depression of nerves the cause of the aura? Functional MRI and other physiological studies of humans with aura suggest that this is the case. If so, aura would therefore be neurological, not vascular.

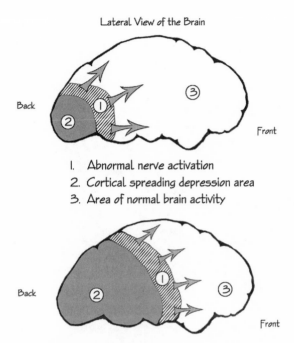

Lateral View of the Brain

Back

Front

1. Abnormal nerve activation
2. Cortical spreading depression area
3. Area of normal brain activity

Back

Front

Fig. 4.1 Cortical Spreading Depression (the cause for aura).

This idea is worth reviewing, because it puts together much of what we have covered so far. An inherited problem in the nerves of the brain causes them to act abnormally and to intermittently fire. Nerves firing in the visual portion of the brain can result in an immediate spreading depression of nerve function in the wake of the activation. This wave of activation, followed by spreading depression and decreased nerve activity, is perceived as slowly moving aura.

The Migraine Generator

The migraine generator was first visualized in 1995. Dr. Hans-Christoph Diener and his associates in Essen, Germany studied men with right-sided migraine without aura. They put these patients in a positron emission tomography (PET) scanner to study what happened during their migraines.

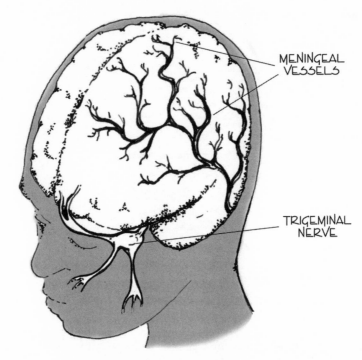

MENINGEAL
VESSELS

TRIGEMINAL
NERVE

Fig. 4.2 Nerve Pathways Leading to Meningeal Blood Vessels.

There appeared to be an area in the lower part of the brain (brain-stem) in which nerve cells turned on at the beginning of the migraine, remained on for the length of the migraine and clicked off at the end of the migraine. Professor H. C. Diener, of Essen, Germany, referred to this center as the *migraine generator* because he believed it to be the area of the brain where the migraine originates. The exact location for the generator may be the dorsal raphe nucleus of the brainstem.

Most functions of the nervous system are controlled by nerves that cross over to the opposite side of the brain. That is true of the migraine generator as well, and only the left brainstem dorsal raphe is turned on in patients with right-sided migraine pain.

The migraine generator only indirectly causes head pain, because it first has to activate a head pain system. The generator connects to nerve pathways that lead to the meninges, coverings around the brain between brain and skull. These pathways lead to other nerves that encircle and serve blood vessels of the meninges. When this occurs, blood vessels in the meninges dilate and the neurons release inflammatory chemicals around the vessels. The combination of meningeal blood vessel dilation and inflammation is believed to be the cause of migraine pain. The dilating vessels could account for the throbbing quality of the pain.

The Trigeminovascular System

The primary problem in migraine, though, is from firing nerves, not from dilating blood vessels (although inflammation may be another cause of the migraine pain). The connection between the migraine generator and the nerves and blood vessels of the meninges is called the *trigeminovascular system*.

To simplify: the migraine central generator clicks on the switch, the trigeminovascular system is activated, the blood vessels of the coverings of the brain dilate, and the meninges become inflamed. The central generator is in the brain and the peripheral pain mechanism in the meninges.

It is not known how an aura with spreading depression turns on the generator, or how the generator turns on in the absence of aura. Perhaps the generator is the major point at which the hyperexcitable nerve cells do their intermittent firing.

Meningitis is also an inflammation of the meninges, but it is usually due to an infection. Migraine pain is like a sterile, non-infectious meningitis, because the meninges become inflamed. And like migraine, meningitis hurts.

Serotonin

Nerves communicate with each other via chemicals that diffuse across space between nerves and turn on the next nerve. These chemicals are called *neurotransmitters*.

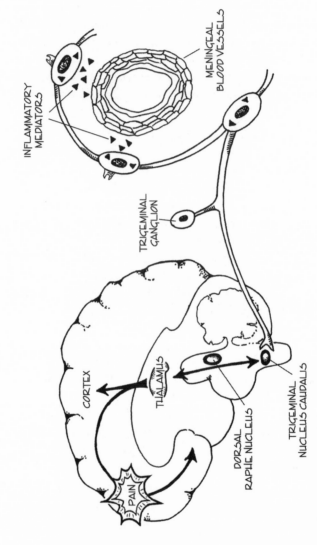

Fig. 4.3 Trigeminovascular System.

Certain nerves release specific chemicals; others receive only signals communicated by those chemicals. In effect, some nerves speak only one language, the language of that particular neurotransmitter. Neurotransmitters can excite or inhibit nerve actions. Some nerve chemicals can do both, depending on where they go in the nervous system, and which nerves they reach. These "ambidextrous neurotransmitters" are like a driver's foot in a car. The foot can work the brake, accelerator, or clutch.

Serotonin is a neurotransmitter that can both excite and inhibit—and therein lies the story of how it controls migraine.

The seven known classes of serotonin nerves in the brain are denoted serotonin 1–7. Serotonin is often abbreviated as 5-HT after its chemical name, 5-hydroxytryptamine. Thus, these are the 5-HT_{1-7} nerves, and the areas on the nerves that receive the serotonin are the 5-HT receptors.

5-HT_1 receptors are negative or inhibitory receptors; 5-HT_2 receptors are positive or excitatory receptors. It is possible that when serotonin binds to the excitatory 5-HT_2 receptors near the migraine central generator, it turns on the migraine. Serotonin 2 may be the switch at the generator or the route to the accelerator.

Migraine patients may have too much release of serotonin at the central generator, or there may be too many accelerators, or the accelerator is too easily depressed. Why the generator turns on only in distinct episodes and in response to particular triggers is one of the mysteries of migraine.

When the generator turns on, it activates the pathways that cause inflammation and blood vessel dilation in the meninges. 5-HT_1 receptors can turn off the inflammation and shrink the vessels. Therefore, to control the 5-HT_1 system is to control the migraine pain. It is like putting the foot on the brake.

Serotonin can act like a foot on the accelerator: if it binds to the 5-HT_2 receptors, it turns on migraine. But serotonin can act like a brake: if it binds to the 5-HT_1 receptors, it turns off the migraine pain, by deactivating the inflammation and shrinking the swollen vessels.

There are two main types of 5-HT_1 receptors, 5-HT_{1B} and 5-HT_{1D}. The 5-HT_{1B} receptor is on the blood vessels of the meninges;

activating it shrinks blood vessels. When it occurs outside the brain, the 5-HT_{1D} receptor turns off the inflammation by preventing the nerves from releasing the chemicals that are the cause. The chemical most likely to have neuroinflammatory effect in migraine is calcitonin gene related peptide, or CGRP, which also dilates blood vessels. Serotonin, activating the 5-HT_{1D} receptor, may help get rid of migraine pain by inhibiting CGRP release.

Therefore, when the serotonin binds to both 5-HT_{1B} and 5-HT_{1D} receptors, both mechanisms of migraine, blood vessel dilation and inflammation, are turned off.

Finally, the signal has to get back into the brain from the inflammation and blood vessel dilation. 5-HT_{1D} receptors in the brain control the portal of entry of the signal from the meninges. If these "central" 5-HT_{1D} receptors are activated, they block the entrance and inhibit the signal's reentry into the brain.

Now we have the whole picture for migraine control. We need to turn off or inhibit 5-HT_2 receptors to prevent the generator from turning on—like keeping the foot off the accelerator—and we need to turn on 5-HT_{1B} and 5-HT_{1D} receptors to turn off the inflammation and shrink the swollen vessels in the meninges and prevent the entry of pain signals into the brain—like stepping on the brake. Many of our best medications for headache can be understood by keeping in mind these mechanisms.

5. Evaluating Migraines

The treatment for migraine depends upon how bad the migraine is, in terms of all of its characteristics. Migraines vary in frequency and in intensity. The severity of the migraine determines how disabled a patient is; establishing the degree of disability leads to the crafting of appropriate treatment.

Migraine treatment should always be at least in part non-pharmacologic—that is, without medications. Medications can be preventive (prophylactic) or as-needed (acute, abortive).

Preventive care means taking a daily medication to prevent the migraines. The U.S. Food and Drug Administration, when evaluating a medication for prevention, looks for whether the medication reduces the frequency of migraine in the majority of the people who take it. It is important to realize that most daily preventive medications do not completely prevent all headaches, and sometimes reduce the intensity or duration of the headaches but not the frequency.

Acute care means taking medication to get rid of the migraine as it occurs. When migraine is not frequent, this may be all that is needed.

So how does a patient decide whether to take medication at all, to take daily preventive medication, or to take medication only as needed? The first step in evaluating headaches is evaluating the severity; the second is evaluating the disability, impact, or time loss suffered.

Evaluating the Severity of Migraines

Several factors are involved in determining the severity of migraine. First, what is the peak intensity? The IHS rates headache pain from 0–3, where 0 is no pain, 1 is mild pain, 2 is moderate pain, and 3 is severe pain.

Second, how fast do the headaches reach peak intensity? Does the patient wake up with them, do they progress explosively in less than 30 minutes, or do they build slowly over several hours?

Third, how bad are the other symptoms of migraine at its peak intensity? Is the patient nauseated or vomiting, or is there photophonophobia or restriction of activity?

Finally, how fast do the associated symptoms reach that level of intensity? How quickly is there nausea? How much time between nausea and vomiting?

To simplify, these four factors help rate the severity of migraines:

1. Peak intensity
2. Time to peak intensity
3. Associated symptoms such as nausea and dislike of light and noise
4. Time to the associated symptoms

Of course, the headache may not be the same each time it occurs, so it is useful to look at the range of the headaches in terms of these characteristics. Knowing the peak of the headache and the time to the peak allows a patient to figure out whether it is appropriate to try to stop the headache with tablet, nasal spray, or injection. If a patient with migraine is nauseated, it may not be such a good idea to take a pill, because in gastric stasis a tablet may not be absorbed very well. In that circumstance, a nasal spray, injection, or suppository may work better or more consistently.

A full list of the questions to evaluate follows:

- How intense are the migraines? Are they mild, moderate, or severe (1, 2, 3)?
- What percentage or fraction of the headaches are mild, moderate, or severe over a month or a year?
- How quickly do they become severe? What is the time between the onset of the headache and the time that the pain is maximal?
- What associated symptoms occur with the headaches—nausea, loss of appetite, vomiting, dislike of light, dislike of noise, dislike of smells?

- How quickly do the associated symptoms develop? For instance, what is the time between the onset of the headache and the development of nausea or vomiting?
- Is the migraine full blown upon waking? Is there nausea or vomiting upon waking? Over a month or a year, what percentage or fraction of the headaches is present upon awakening, and what fraction develops during the day?

Headache Diaries or Calendars

Another way to evaluate the need for treatment is to document the frequency of the migraines. A headache diary or calendar is very useful for documenting when and how often headaches and their other characteristics occur.

Many aspects of migraines can be put into the diary, but the minimum information is the dates of the headaches and their intensity. Diaries can also record triggers for headache, the dates of the menstrual period, how each headache was treated, and how well the treatment worked.

Evaluating Headache Disability

Two relatively easy tests can be used to establish the disability or impact of migraines. The first is the Migraine Disability Assessment Test (MIDAS), a series of questions developed by Drs. Lipton and Stewart.

The MIDAS Test

1. On how many days in the last three months did you miss work or school because of your headaches?
2. On how many days in the last three months was your productivity at work or school reduced by half or more because of your headaches? (Do not include days counted in question 1.)

| Day | Time | | Severity * | Other symptoms | Medication 1 | | | Medication 2 | | | Possible Triggers |
	Onset	End			Name	Dose	Relief**	Name	Dose	Relief**	

*Scale of 0–3: no pain 0; pain as bad as it can be 3
**Scale of 0–3: no relief 0; complete relief 3

Fig. 5.1 Migraine Calendar.

3. On how many days in the last three months did you not do household work because of your headaches?
4. On how many days in the last three months was your productivity in household work reduced by half or more because of your headaches? (Do not include days counted in question 3.)
5. On how many days in the last three months did you miss family, social or leisure activities because of your headaches?

The Headache Impact Test (HIT) can be found at www. headachetest.com and www.amIhealthy.com. HIT is a "dynamic" test, meaning that the next question administered is determined by the answer to the previous question. This allows the test to be crafted for a specific person, and geared to the level of that person's headaches.

HIT averages about five questions, the same as MIDAS; however, HIT chooses the five questions from over 50 possibilities. A patient can take the test at home, print the results, and bring them when going to the doctor. The results tell about how much time per month patients with similar headaches are losing.

The HIT-6 is a paper version of the online HIT that uses the six most sensitive and specific questions.

If a patient can show a caregiver how much time is being lost, it is possible that the caregiver will pay more attention to his or her headaches. And that should lead to more appropriate and aggressive treatment for the patient. It has been shown that patients with high impact, disability, or time loss from migraines do better if given migraine-specific treatment (triptans) initially than if given non-specific treatment (e.g. analgesics).

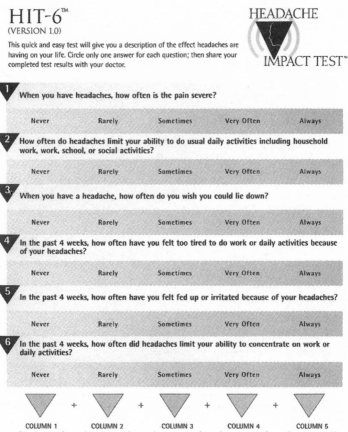

Fig. 5.2 Headache Impact Test.

What does your score mean?

If you scored 60+

Your headaches are having a very severe impact on your life. You may be experiencing disabling pain and other symptoms that are more severe than those of other headache sufferers. Don't let your headaches stop you from enjoying the important things in your life, like family, work, school or social activities.

Make an appointment *today* to discuss your HIT-6 results and your headaches with your doctor.

If you scored 56–58

Your headaches are having a substantial impact on your life. As a result you may be experiencing severe pain and other symptoms, causing you to miss some time from family, work, school or social activities.

Make an appointment *today* to discuss your HIT-6 results and your headaches with your doctor.

If you scored 50–54

Your headaches seem to be having some impact on your life. Your headaches should not make you miss time from family, work, school or social activities.

Make sure you discuss your HIT-6 results and your headaches at your next appointment with your doctor.

If you scored 48 or less

Your headaches seem to be having little to no impact on your life at this time. We encourage you to take HIT-6 monthly to continue to track how your headaches affect your life.

About HIT

The Headache Impact Test (HIT) is a tool used to measure the impact headaches have on your ability to function on the job, at school, at home and in social situations.

Your score shows you the effect that headaches have on normal daily life and your ability to function.

HIT is not intended to offer medical advice regarding medical diagnosis or treatment. You should talk to your healthcare provider for advice specific to your situation.

If your score on HIT-6 is 50 or higher, you should share the results with your doctor. Headaches that are disrupting your life could be migraine.

HIT was developed by an international team of headache experts from neurology and primary care medicine in collaboration with the psychometricians who developed the SF-36** health assessment tool.

HIT is also available on the Internet at www.headachetest.com.

The Internet version allows you to print out a personal report of your results as well as a special detailed version for your doctor.

SF-36 is a registered trademark of Medical Outcomes Trust and John E. Ware, Jr.

Take HIT-6 with you when you visit your doctor because research shows that when doctors understand exactly how badly headaches affect the lives of their patients, they are much more likely to provide a successful treatment program, which may include medication.

Don't forget to take HIT-6 again or try the Internet version at www.headachetest.com to continue to monitor your progress.

HEADACHE IMPACT TEST™

Fig. 5.2 (*continued*).

6. Acute Treatment of Migraine

How to Judge Medications that Turn Off Headache

How does one tell how well a medication works to eliminate a migraine? Researchers and doctors use many measures in evaluating as-needed, acute treatments that stop a migraine attack. The FDA then uses the results of testing of medications on these measures to determine efficacy.

In older studies on acute medications, patients were required to wait to treat until their migraine reached moderate to severe levels of pain. In real life, patients usually treat early, when their pain is mild, as soon as they know that a migraine is developing. Since the medications are studied in treatment of more advanced attacks at higher levels of pain, the estimate of effectiveness of treatment included in prescribing information is lower than patients can expect when they treat earlier with lower levels of pain.

There are a number ways of rating how effectively a migraine medication gets rid of a headache. One is to measure headache response, which is also called headache relief or pain relief. Headache response means that a medication takes a headache from moderate to severe intensity (that is, from number 2–3 to 3) down to no headache or mild headache (0–1 to 3).

One problem with headache response is that it does not measure what most patients want most, which is to be pain free after taking a medication. If a moderate migraine is treated, and the medication only takes the pain down to a mild level, the patient may describe this as only "taking the edge off the pain." Also, headache response is measured within a specified amount of time, such as one, two, or four hours. Obviously, if someone has a fast building migraine, waiting four hours is too long to get relief from a drug.

A measurement more in line with migraine patient wishes is pain free. Pain free measures what percentage of patients gets to no headache at all within a particular amount of time, conventionally by two hours.

The speed with which a medication works can be evaluated in a number of ways. One is to see at what point a significant number of patients have pain relief or are pain free. Another is to measure the "time to headache relief" and the "time to pain free."

Finally, it is useful to measure whether a medication effect lasts. Once someone has pain relief or is pain free, does the same headache come back within 24 hours? This can be a big problem with certain anti-migraine drugs. When a person gets pain relief but the same headache does return within 24 hours, this is called *headache recurrence*. Recurrence is measured as a percentage of patients treated with a headache medication who get relief and then return of the headache within 24 hours.

Low-level Medication Treatment

Moderate to high intensity, time loss, or disability merits migraine-specific treatment. Low-level headaches can be ameliorated with non-specific treatment.

As is true for all acute treatment, the trick to making migraine medication work is to get the medication in at the earliest glimmer of the migraine, earlier than early. Obviously, low-level medication will not work if a person wakes up with a migraine, or if the migraine gallops—that is, develops very rapidly.

The patient may not be severely disabled by low-level migraine, and if the attack is treated very early, low-level treatment can work. Most of these medications are available without prescription, and all are inexpensive. Most people with low-level migraine do not seek medical attention, because they do not usually experience disability, and can treat effectively with over-the-counter medication.

Naproxen sodium can stop or abort a migraine in doses as low as 220 mg, the over-the-counter strength (Aleve), or as high as 825 mg. Other nonsteroidal anti-inflammatory drugs can also work, including ibuprofen (Advil), ketoprofen (Orudis), and aspirin. Perhaps they work by preventing the inflammation that occurs in the meninges; however, the significance of the inflammation that accompanies migraine is hotly debated and may not be the significant cause for the pain.

Recent studies have shown that two Excedrin (each of which contains 250 mg of aspirin, 250 mg of acetaminophen [Tylenol], and 65 mg of caffeine) can abort low-level migraine. How each of these components works in migraine is not known. Extra Strength Excedrin and Excedrin Migraine are identical products with different packaging.

Medium-level Medication Treatment

Like low-level treatments, medium-level treatments are non-specific. Moderate migraine medications require a prescription but are quite inexpensive. Unlike the triptans that will be discussed later, medium-level medications do not turn on the serotonin receptors that turn off migraine, but they can work on non-disabling migraine if the conditions are right: the migraine has to develop during the day, it has to develop relatively slowly, and it cannot be a severe migraine. Studies have shown that if a person has disability or time loss of even 50% from migraines, trying low- or medium-level medication first is not a good strategy. The presence of significant time loss or impact means that migraine-specific medications such as triptans, used from the beginning, will result in better outcome and lower cost.

The mildest medium-level combination prescription medication is a mixture of isometheptene, acetaminophen, and chlorzoxazone (Midrin). The isometheptene is a mild blood vessel constrictor; the chlorzoxazone is a mild tranquilizer or muscle relaxer; and the acetaminophen (Tylenol) is a mild analgesic, although not an anti-inflammatory. As with Excedrin, it is unknown how this combination works.

The next step up in strength is the mixture of butalbital, a barbiturate, with other medications. It can be mixed with caffeine and aspirin (Fiorinal) or caffeine and acetaminophen (Fioricet, Esgic Plus). Codeine can be added (Fiorinal #3, Fioricet #3), or the caffeine can be excluded (Phrenilin, Axotal). Once again, the triad mixture contains a mild blood vessel constrictor (caffeine), tranquilizer or muscle relaxer (butalbital), and mild pain killer (aspirin or acetaminophen, with or without codeine). Everything true of Midrin is true of Fiorinal—it has to be taken early (one or two at onset) and, although it can cause drowsiness or agitation in some patients, it is usually without side effects.

Stronger still are medications that contain narcotic painkillers, or opioids. All of these can get rid of low-level migraine, and most are mixed with aspirin or acetaminophen. The lower potency the opioid, the less likely it is to cause drowsiness. Low-level opioids include tramadol (Ultram), propoxyphene (Darvon), codeine, which when mixed with acetaminophen is called Tylenol #3, and hydrocodone, which when mixed with acetaminophen is called Vicodin or Lorcet. Instructions for use and side effects are the same as with Midrin and Fiorinal.

All of the low- and medium-level medications share a risk of habituation. This is especially true with Fiorinal and opioid-containing medications. I recommend that people with non-disabling migraine use lower or moderate level mixed headache medications no more than two days per week, to avoid dependence—and that even lower frequency of use is better. I rarely, if ever, initiate these treatments because patients in neurology or primary care offices complaining of headache almost always have disabling migraine and so should be prescribed triptans.

When a patient starts using these medications too often, it is usually time to place that patient onto a daily preventive medication, to reduce both the frequency of migraines and the use of the acute, as-needed medications.

The reason for my recommendation for infrequent use of low- and medium-level medications is not my concern that a patient will get addicted, in the usual sense. Rather, migraine patients can transform from discrete episodes of migraine into daily headache when the use of these medications climbs to three or more days of treatment per week. When the wearing off of the medication seems to trigger the next headache on a daily or near daily basis, it is called *rebound headache* (see chapter 8).

It is extremely important to conclude these sections on nonspecific medication with a discussion of three strategies for treatment. *Step care across attacks* is the strategy of starting with a non-specific treatment for several attacks, and switching to a migraine-specific treatment (triptan) if low- or medium-level treatments do not work after several attacks. *Step care within attacks* means starting with a non-specific treatment and rescuing with a triptan if low-level treatment fails on that attack.

Neither of these approaches works very well. *Stratified care* is defined as matching patient or attack characteristics to treatment from the beginning. Use of time loss, impact, or disability as a marker for migraine severity is a shortcut to deciding appropriate treatment. It has been shown that, if there are 11 or more days in the last three months of at least 50% time loss from work, home, school, or recreational activity due to headache, use of low- or medium-level treatment rather than migraine-specific treatment results in worse outcomes, greater time loss, and greater costs—and that almost all patients complaining of headache in a primary care office have significantly disabling migraine.

It is therefore not a good strategy to seek inexpensive, nonspecific treatment if migraines have impact. Rather, migraine-specific treatment such as triptans should be used to stop attacks and taken early without temporizing.

Migraine-Specific Treatments

Ergots

Migraine-specific medications are used in migraines that cause disability, are severe in some way, or do not respond to lower level treatment. The grandparents of modern migraine designer medications are the ergots.

Ergots are derivatives of a rye mold, *Claviceps purpurea*. This mold that commonly grew on bread in the Middle Ages can cause hallucinations ("St. Anthony's fire") and blood vessel constriction in the fingers. It is now known that the mold also can cause uterine contractions.

Ergots are serotonin-active drugs. They activate many serotonin receptors, most of which turn off migraine, but some of which turn on migraine and nausea. The most important of the anti-migraine effects come from the 5-HT_{1B} and 5-HT_{1D} receptors. Ergots turn on 5-HT_{1B} receptors in the blood vessels covering the brain, and shrink the swollen vessels activated in migraine. Ergots constrict blood vessels all over the body.

They also activate the 5-HT_{1D} receptors. This results in reducing the inflammation in the meninges associated with migraine. Activating 5-HT_{1D} receptors in the brainstem also interferes with transmission of the pain signal, and inhibits nausea.

Ergotamine tartrate

In the nineteenth century, pulverized ergot mold was sometimes injected intravenously to help expel the placenta after birth. The Swiss chemist Arthur Stoll isolated the active ingredient of the ergot mold in 1918. This was ergotamine tartrate, which is the active ingredient in Cafergot.

Ergotamine was initially used for gynecologic care but proved to be useful for migraine. It is tricky to use, however; it is not well absorbed in pill form, and therefore has been available in other forms. Ergotamine is available as injection and nasal spray in some countries, but not the U.S.

In the U.S., it is available as a rectal suppository, Cafergot, which is the most reliable but least socially acceptable way to take it.

It is also available in oral tablets, but only about 3% is absorbed in this form, so its reliability and usefulness is limited. Ergotamine and caffeine are mixed in a coated tablet (Cafergot, Ercaf), which is coated so the pill cannot be cut. Many people get nauseated from a full dose of ergotamine and require a lower dose, and currently there are no breakable tablets available in the U.S., so pill usage of ergotamine has plummeted. When ergotamine is tolerated, about a third of patients can obtain pain relief within two hours from the mixture of oral ergotamine and caffeine.

Bellergal is ergotamine mixed with a barbiturate tranquilizer, phenobarbital, and a belladonna-like medication, a derivative of the poison made from deadly nightshade and used by the Borgias in the Renaissance. There are very few reasons to mix in either medication with ergotamine, so this is rarely prescribed.

Ergotamine has the potential for many side effects. As noted, it can cause nausea. It narrows all arteries, those in the extremities and those in the heart and brain.

There is a condition in which cold induces ischemia of the digits. The tips of the fingers and toes turn white, then blue, and sometimes red. It can be dramatic. This condition is called Raynaud's phenomenon.

Raynaud's is more common in migraine patients. (Migraine patients also tend to have cold hands and feet, which is different from true Raynaud's with its clear color changes.) Ergotamine worsens Raynaud's badly, and can cause the small arteries in fingers and toes to go into spasm. This can lead to gangrene. Thus, ergotamine should not be used in people with Raynaud's syndrome.

Ergots, including ergotamine, narrow coronary arteries by 20% in normal people at therapeutic doses. The narrowing persists for days. This narrowing means that there are some very important limitations to the use of ergotamine.

For example, some people have a tendency to have arterial spasm. In particular, they can get spasm of the arteries in the heart, and chest pain (angina) from the spasm, rather than from clogging of the arteries (atherosclerosis). The spasm-caused angina is called Prinzmetal angina. It occurs with greater frequency in migraine patients, although still quite infrequently. Ergotamine can precipitate the coronary arterial spasm or Prinzmetal angina, and so cannot be used by people with Prinzmetal syndrome.

Spasm of coronary arteries is more likely if there is atherosclerosis; and if the coronary artery is three-quarters clogged and the ergotamine narrows coronaries by 10–20%, a person is at risk of a heart attack or sudden death. For that reason, ergotamine should not be used in people with coronary artery disease.

Frequent use of ergotamine can cause arteries to remain in spasm, and arms and legs can get cold and achy. This is called ergotism, and is dangerous. The arms and legs can suffer permanent damage from the decreased blood flow, and this can lead to tissue death and gangrene.

There is a rare side effect of long-term, repetitive use of ergotamine (that also occurs occasionally with other rye mold ergot medications) in which scar tissue can develop on heart valves, or on the coverings of the heart, in the lungs, or in the gut. This is called fibrosis, and can also occur where the ergotamine is used. For example, if ergotamine is overused as a suppository, rectal scar tissue can form and even close off the rectum.

Frequent use of ergotamine is also habit forming. People with migraine are particularly susceptible to using ergotamine too often. If ergotamine is used more than two times per week, an ergot habit can be created, called ergot habituation.

Habituation to ergotamine is a serious problem for people with migraine. Once a migraine sufferer begins to overuse ergotamine, the frequency of the headaches increases until the headaches become (and ergotamine use is) daily or near daily. This rebound is also called *transformed or chronic migraine with medication overuse* and will be discussed further in chapter 8.

Habituation to ergotamine causes one of the worst forms of rebound. Every time the ergot-habituated person tries to stop the ergotamine, a severe headache caused by the withdrawal of the ergotamine ensues. To make matters worse, once a patient is habituated to ergotamine, neither preventive medications for migraine nor other as-needed medications will work for headache. The rebound medication, the ergotamine, nullifies the effect of other medications.

Almost no one habituated to ergotamine can break the cycle and get free of the repetitive use of this medication without medical help, usually in the hospital. So it is very important to limit the use of ergotamine to no more than once weekly, and if possible less frequently than that.

Given that this is a difficult medication to use, and perilous to overuse, when should ergotamine be prescribed? The answer has to do with some of the special properties of the ergotamine.

Ergotamine has long action, and once it works, the migraine has very little chance of recurring, although the reasons for this are not known. It is difficult to get the ergotamine absorbed at an adequate dose without nausea. It is important to find the maximal dose of ergotamine that does not cause nausea, and then use that dose when the migraine hits.

Ergotamine cannot be given as a prescription dose and then, without preparation, tried in an acute attack. A patient really has to try it in advance and figure out the right dose. If the ergotamine is used at too high a dose and causes nausea, the migraine usually gets worse, so it is important to get the right dose.

There are several ways to do this. Only if there is no vomiting early in the migraine can oral ergotamine be used. I tell my patients to try an oral ergotamine and see if they tolerate when they do not have a migraine.

If the patient cannot tolerate oral ergotamine, it becomes necessary to use the Cafergot suppository. Again, it is necessary to try out the suppository in advance, before using it in an attack, and find the biggest dose that does not cause nausea. Since the suppository is better absorbed than the pills, the drug works more effectively and more consistently by this route, and often at a much lower dose.

In conclusion, ergotamine, with its long action, can be used in long-lasting migraine (such as menstrual migraine) to avoid the migraine recurring. But it is crucial to establish the dose in advance to avoid nausea, and to limit ergotamine use to once weekly, preferably less often. Also, ergotamine should not be taken by pregnant women.

Given all of these prerequisites and the potential side effects of the drug, ergotamine use has decreased and has been replaced with newer, safer, and more effective designer medications (triptans) to treat migraine on an as-needed basis. Despite this fact, some HMOs and insurance plans in many parts of the U.S. still insist on doctors prescribing ergotamine before these newer drugs, because ergotamine is less expensive. It should be clear from the above discussion that requiring prescriptions of ergotamine based on cost and without consideration of toxicity is being penny wise and pound foolish.

Dihydroergotamine mesylate (DHE)

Dihydroergotamine (DHE) is another derivative of rye mold, but is an improvement over ergotamine. It is less nauseating, less habit forming, and causes less constriction of the vessels in the arms and legs.

However, a recent study from the Netherlands found that DHE causes just as much narrowing of coronary arteries as ergotamine, and likewise should not be used with coronary artery disease or Prinzmetal angina.

DHE is also very poorly absorbed orally. It is available as a pill in Europe but not in the U.S. In the U.S., DHE comes in an injectable form called D.H.E. 45, and as a nasal spray called Migranal.

Migranal DHE nasal spray works in about 50% of people in providing headache relief within two hours, and about 60% within four hours. The migraine recurs only about 15% of the time.

The biggest problems with the nasal spray are nasal stuffiness in some patients and a cumbersome preparation in order to use it. The current kit requires a user to break a glass ampoule, load a sprayer device, prime it, spray once in both nostrils, and repeat the sprays in 15 minutes. Nausea is far less of a problem with the DHE nasal spray than with ergotamine.

The DHE injection is very effective. It can be administered sub-cutaneously, intramuscularly, and intravenously. When a migraine goes on and on, and nothing seems to work, intravenous DHE can be used to terminate it. I usually give an anti-nausea medication before administering intravenous DHE.

People habituated to medications and in rebound with chronic daily headache can actually be detoxified using DHE. Patients are hospitalized and put on preventive migraine medication. The medication causing the rebound, even ergotamine, is discontinued, and intravenous anti-nausea medication and intravenous DHE are administered every eight hours. The patient goes through withdrawal, but the intravenous DHE helps with the withdrawal headache. As many as 92% of people are headache-free in three days.

Patients can be taught to use self-injections of DHE at home. Since DHE stings when injected, I teach them to mix it with the anesthetic lidocaine. They draw up the lidocaine and the DHE in the same syringe using a tiny subcutaneous needle, and then self-inject.

DHE does not come with an autoinjector. It must be self-administered the old-fashioned way.

DHE is cumbersome to use, involves needles and syringes, can be nauseating, and sometimes requires individualized dosage adjustment. But in comparison to ergotamine, DHE is better tolerated in that it causes less nausea, less limb artery constriction, and less frequent fibrosis. It works in a higher percentage of patients, it has an equally low likelihood of the headache recurring, and it is far less habit-forming than ergotamine.

Some women use DHE for long menstrual migraines because of its low recurrence rate. It too is absolutely contraindicated in pregnancy.

Other ergots

The same rye mold is the source of many medications. Some, such as bromocriptine (Parlodel) and pergolide (Permax), are used to treat Parkinson disease. Others, like methylergonovine (Methergine), are used to stop uterine bleeding after birth.

The most infamous of all ergots is LSD. It works by binding irreversibly to serotonin receptors in the brain, which makes people dream while awake. This accounts for the hallucinations that occur when people use LSD. The chemical differences between the clinically used ergots and LSD are small.

Some oral ergots are used daily on a preventive basis for migraine (see chapter 7). Methylergonovine can be used this way.

Triptans

The big revolution in migraine in the past 15 years has been the development of migraine-specific medications, the triptans. Their discovery was due to the persistence of Patrick Humphrey and his research team at the pharmaceutical company Glaxo, Inc. Humphrey and his colleagues set out to create serotonin-active medications. After more than a decade of work, they synthesized sumatriptan in 1984.

All triptans share certain basic characteristics. Like ergots, they activate $5\text{-}HT_{1B}$ receptors and constrict meningeal blood vessels that become activated in migraine. Also like ergots, they turn on $5\text{-}HT_{1D}$ receptors and eliminate inflammation in the meninges and transmission of pain signals in the brain itself. Triptans have not been found to stop aura and the migraine that follows, though patients who get aura benefit by waiting until the aura is over and then taking their triptan at the earliest onset of pain, preferably when the pain is mild.

It is always hard to compare headache medications, and many factors need to be considered in choosing the appropriate triptan. For example, should we compare the speed of pain relief, whether the patient becomes pain free, or the likelihood of remaining without headache after successful treatment—that is, no recurrence? What if the triptan works well but is inconsistent, and there is no assurance it will work most of the time? Or if it works well but has unacceptable side effects? The following questions provide a useful guide for evaluating the different triptans:

1. What forms and doses are available? Does it come as a pill, shot, nasal spray, melt (an oral tablet that dissolves in the mouth, is swallowed, and then absorbed like a pill)? Are there several dosage strengths?
2. How fast does the drug reach a maximum concentration in the blood? How long does it take for the medication to leave the body? Is the medication eliminated by the liver or kidney, and by what chemical systems?
3. How fast does the medication take effect?

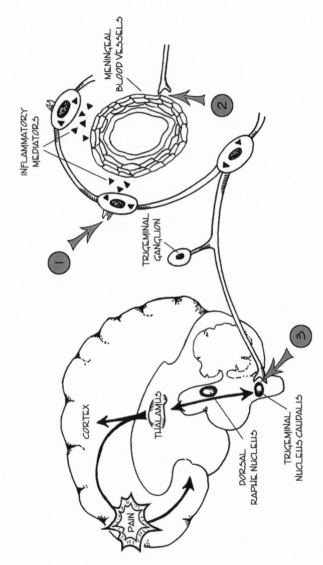

Fig. 6.1 Triptan Mechanisms for Migraine.

4. What is the likelihood of pain relief or headache response within two hours?
5. What is the likelihood of becoming pain free within two hours?
6. What is the likelihood that the same migraine will recur within 24 hours after pain relief has been achieved with the medication?
7. What is the consistency of the medication with long-term use?
8. What are the side effects of the medication?
9. How does this particular triptan stack up against the others?
10. What is the maximum amount allowed per 24 hours?

Deciding how to judge effectiveness is not a trivial issue. Many people who do not respond to one medication will respond to another. Many people strongly prefer one triptan to another.

The true answer to the question of whether one triptan is superior to another is answered by how well it works for the individual. And it is well worth trying another triptan if the first one tried does not work satisfactorily or has unacceptable side effects.

There are a few important points to bear in mind when considering a switch from one triptan to another. It has been shown that some people who do not respond to a triptan on the first try may respond on a second or third separate migraine. So I tell my patients not to give up on a triptan until they have tried it on three separate attacks. Remember that trying a triptan three times means on three separate migraines, not three times in one attack.

A second point to remember is that there are many ways that a triptan can fail to work. The triptan can have an inadequate speed of onset. It may get rid of a headache but take longer to work. Or the triptan can take the migraine from moderate or severe down to mild, but not to zero. Although this is considered pain relief, it can be inadequate, and many people consider relief without being pain free a lack of treatment success.

The triptan can be inconsistent in its response. That is, a person can find that it works well on one attack, but not on another. All of the fast acting triptans work on about 80% of attacks. So I tell my patients that, if the triptan is working about 80% of the time, that is about as good as it is going to get, and the triptan should not be switched.

To maximize the likelihood of success with a triptan, maximize the likelihood of becoming pain free, and minimize the risk of recurrence, it is crucial to treat the migraine early. It is not a good idea to "stage" a migraine or treat as step care within attacks. That is, it is self-defeating to try a low-level treatment first with an attack and then use the triptan as rescue only if the lower level treatment fails.

The triptan always works better when taken earlier in the course of the migraine. If the patient waits for the first medication to fail, that reduces the likelihood of success with the triptan, increasing the likelihood of recurrence, and decreasing the consistency of response. One reason a given triptan may be inconsistent in getting rid of a headache is that a person may take it at different times during the attack, with differing results.

Some people feel that the recurrence or return of the headache is a failure of the drug. So they feel that even if the medication works fast, and completely restores normal function, it is still a failure if the headache comes back in 12 hours. However, all the triptans, and indeed all headache-relieving medications, are associated with some recurrence. If a patient has success with no recurrence with a given triptan, the triptan should not be switched.

Finally, although there is not a lot of difference in the oral fast-acting triptans in terms of side effects, some people clearly get side effects from one but not with another.

The two groups of triptans

All triptans were not created equal. Triptans can be divided roughly into two groups.

Group I consists of sumatriptan (Imitrex), zolmitriptan (Zomig), rizatriptan (Maxalt), almotriptan (Axert), and eletriptan (Relpax). These have relatively fast onset of action, with over 60% of people getting pain relief within two hours. However, there is generally at least a 30% chance that the same headache will recur after taking these medications for a moderate to severe level intensity headache.

Some patients do not mind repeating a dose if the headache recurs; they are most interested in rapid onset of significant benefit from a medication that stops migraine in its tracks. Other patients do not mind waiting longer for a medication to take effect, knowing that once it works the headache will not recur.

Group II consists of naratriptan (Amerge) and frovatriptan (Frova). Like ergots, specifically ergotamine and DHE, this group is associated with slow onset of effect but low chance of recurrence of the headache. With these triptans it takes up to four hours for about 60% of people to get headache relief. However, the likelihood of the headache coming back is definitely lower with naratriptan, only occurring about 20% of the time, and probably lower with frovatriptan.

Triptan side effects

Like ergots, all triptans narrow coronary arteries by 10–20% and so should not be used by people with coronary artery disease. Unlike ergots, the constriction of coronary arteries caused by triptans goes away rapidly. For the overwhelming number of patients, the narrowing causes no symptoms, and the risk of serious heart cardiotoxicity is very, very low.

Because vascular constriction can occur, doctors evaluate patients for the safety of triptan use. Known risk factors for heart disease include elevated cholesterol, high blood pressure, family history of early heart disease, being overweight, having diabetes, smoking, and being a postmenopausal woman or a man over 40 years old. When multiple risk factors are present, some doctors do a cardiac check on a patient before administering the first triptan dose. When one or fewer risk factors for heart disease are present, usually no work-up is done.

The risks for triptan use, as noted above, are very low. The same evaluation should probably be done for ergots, which have more prolonged coronary artery narrowing, and may be more dangerous. Yet most doctors do not do a cardiac work-up before using ergots, while the work-up before triptan use is often excessive. Serious cardiac events occur with triptans at a rate of less than one in a million—a lower rate than for those that occur with auto accidents or with antibiotics.

All triptans can cause what are referred to as "triptan sensations." These particularly include symptoms of tightening of the jaw, neck, or chest, which are probably due to narrowing of the esophagus caused by the drugs and not related to coronary artery changes. People can also experience tingling, flushing sensations, dizziness, and nausea. These side effects are not dangerous and are at most an annoyance. Almost all of these symptoms occur less frequently when the medication is taken early and become less severe with time.

There is a warning on triptans suggesting that they should be used with caution in people who are taking selective serotonin reuptake inhibitor antidepressants (SSRIs). These include fluoxetine (Prozac), sertraline (Zoloft), paroxetine (Paxil), citalopram (Celexa), venlafaxine (Effexor), nefazadone (Serzone), and fluvoxamine (Luvox).

This is based on the very rare "serotonin syndrome," which occurs when a person with unusual sensitivity to the effects of serotonin takes multiple medications, all of which have serotonin effects in the brain and/or raise the amount of serotonin in the brain. Symptoms include confusion, agitation, tremors and muscle jerks, clumsy walking and incoordination, and even seizures. There have been a very few cases reported of people who may have developed this syndrome when combining an SSRI and a triptan. However, the syndrome is so rare that most patients can use triptans while taking SSRIs without difficulty.

Triptan Group I
Our description of triptans begins with the fast-acting, high-powered triptans with higher recurrence in Group I.

Sumatriptan (Imitrex)
Sumatriptan (Imitrex), the first triptan synthesized, is the most used and most studied triptan. Used by nearly 13 million people to treat about 300 million attacks, it is available in the U.S. in three forms: subcutaneous injection, nasal spray, and oral tablet.

Table 6.1 The Group I triptans – fast acting triptans with higher recurrence

Drug	Brand name	Form	Dose (mg)	Directions
Sumatriptan	Imitrex	Tablet	25, 50, 100	Can repeat in 2 h, maximum 200 mg/24 h
		Subcutaneous injection	6	Can repeat in 1 h, maximum 2 shots/24 h
		Nasal spray	5, 20 (20 is optimum dose)	Can repeat in 2 h, maximum 2 sprays/24 h
Zolmitriptan	Zomig	Tablet, melt	2.5, 5	Can repeat in 2 h, maximum 10 mg/24 h
		Nasal spray	5	
Rizatriptan	Maxalt	Tablet, melt	5, 10 (10 is optimum dose, 5 if on propranolol)	Can repeat in 2 h, maximum 30 mg/24 h, 15 mg/24 h if on propranalol
Almotriptan	Axert	Tablet	12.5	can repeat in 2 h, maximum 25 mg/24 h
Eletriptan	Relpax	Tablet	40	Can repeat in 2 h, maximum 80 mg/24 h

Sumatriptan is a short-lasting medication; half of it is eliminated from the body in about two hours. This is both an advantage and a disadvantage. It means if the patient does not like the drug or its side effects, its effects do not last too long. But even if he or she does like it and it gets rid of the headache rapidly, there is about a 30% chance that the same headache will recur within 24 hours, unless the patient takes the medicine early.

All triptans are eliminated from the body at least partly by the liver. Sumatriptan is metabolized entirely in the liver, almost all of it degraded by the monoamine oxidase (MAO) enzymes. Use of sumatriptan, rizatriptan, and zolmitriptan, all of which have MAO degradation, is contraindicated with the MAO-inhibitors (MAOIs) used to treat depression and, in severe cases, to prevent migraine.

Injectable sumatriptan was the first triptan in any form released in the U.S. It is available for self-administration in a "statdose." Presently, the statdose injector allows the patient to load the sumatriptan injections two to a cartridge, with simple cartridges in which the needle is never seen. A small penlike device is filled with one injection and the sumatriptan is delivered under the skin with a gentle click. This is similar to the popular "epi-pen" that allows for injection of epinephrine in an allergic reaction. The entire unit can fit in a breast pocket.

Subcutaneous sumatriptan sets the standard for speed and effectiveness with triptans. It works rapidly, with 50% of patients getting headache relief within 30 minutes, more than 75% within one hour after treatment, and over 80% experiencing headache relief within two hours. For the 30% of patients who have a recurrence the same day, another dose is safe and effective.

Sumatriptan nasal spray can be as fast as the injection for some people: almost 40% have headache relief within 30 minutes. The spray comes in a single-use device. Unfortunately, when sniffed it frequently causes an unpleasant taste in the back of the throat. For this reason, it is now recommended to spray once in one nostril and not sniff it. The device is then discarded.

The sumatriptan oral tablet is available in the U.S. as 25, 50, and 100 mg tablets. When taken early, the 100 mg dose may yield a greater likelihood of sustained pain freedom than lower doses.

At the end of 2003 a new rapid release tablet took the place of the old tablets, and this new form of pill appears to work much faster than the previous tablet.

All three forms of sumatriptan reduce migraine symptoms such as nausea and dislike of light and noise at essentially the same rate as headache pain. With these different forms, how does a patient decide what to use, and why do we need the different forms?

Some people wake up with their migraine full blown and vomiting. Patients who are vomiting cannot very well take a pill and expect to hold it down long enough to have it take effect, so they will need to use an injection or a nasal spray.

If the migraine is full blown, that patient will want the fastest and most powerful anti-migraine medication there is, and that is the injection of sumatriptan. It has more side effects, is more expensive than a pill or spray, and it is not everyone's cup of tea to take an injection, but it is extraordinarily effective. Subcutaneous sumatriptan truly restores people to normal function, even when the migraine is at the vomiting stage, and many migraine patients always keep the shot around for emergencies.

The FDA has stated that a patient needs to separate taking two different triptans by 24 hours. However, a great advantage of sumatriptan is the flexibility that allows people to use a mixture of forms in the same day; for instance, a patient can use one spray and one injection since they are roughly equivalent. If the patient begins with one form of sumatriptan, such as a pill, and it is not strong enough for a particular migraine, it is acceptable to switch to another form (e.g., the spray or injection) within an hour or two or within the same day.

Not everyone responds to every triptan. Some patients will find relief with sumatriptan by trying it on multiple attacks. It has been shown that sometimes it takes a trial of sumatriptan on three successive migraines to get the benefit.

Sumatriptan is very consistent in its effectiveness for patients who respond to it. One way to measure consistency is to ask what percentage of attacks the drug stops over a year of use. An average of 70–80% of attacks can be stopped within two hours with the three forms.

To summarize, sumatriptan is remarkably effective, flexible, consistent, and safe. It has revolutionized the treatment of an acute migraine. The multiple forms and reliability give the power to stop variable attacks to the patient.

Zolmitriptan (Zomig)

One of the first successors to sumatriptan to be synthesized was zolmitriptan (Zomig). Zolmitriptan has a higher oral absorption rate than sumatriptan and a higher fat solubility, for penetration of the brain.

Zolmitriptan is available as a nasal spray, a tablet, and as an orally dissolvable tablet, or melt (ZMT). This orange flavored melt dissolves in the mouth without water and is absorbed in the stomach. A melt is not a sublingual pill like nitroglycerin. Its effectiveness is virtually identical to that of the traditional tablet, but the melt may be more convenient.

The zolmitriptan tablet reaches maximal concentration in the blood in around two hours. About half of the drug is eliminated from the body within three hours. Like sumatriptan, zolmitriptan is entirely removed from the body by the liver. As with sumatriptan, the MAO system is one of the enzymes that breaks down the zolmitriptan, contraindicating the use of MAOIs.

When using zolmitriptan, most people start with the 2.5 mg pill. About 64% of patients will obtain pain relief and about 24% are pain free by two hours with the 2.5 mg dose. By four hours, 72% of patients have headache relief and 42% are pain free. After the successful treatment of headache, about 30% of the time the pain recurs.

The 5 mg pill is more likely than the 2.5 mg pill to make people pain free within two hours, with 36% pain free. However, the 5 mg dose has more side effects than the 2.5 mg dose. These side effects are the usual triptan sensations.

Two out of three studies directly comparing zolmitriptan and sumatriptan failed to show clinically significant differences between the two. Zolmitriptan tablets do not work faster than sumatriptan tablets, and there is no real difference in side effects.

The new 5 mg nasal spray works more rapidly than a tablet with onset of effect as early as 5 minutes and 70% of patients getting relief within two hours. Over a year, zolmitriptan yielded pain relief in about 80% of attacks by two hours with a single dose in people who respond to it.

Rizatriptan (Maxalt)
Rizatriptan is available in two oral forms, a regular tablet and a mint-tasting melt. As with sumatriptan and zolmitriptan, rizatriptan is broken down in the liver by MAO and is contraindicated with MAOIs.

In four studies the traditional 10 mg dose resulted in two-hour headache response or pain relief ranging from 67–77%. Two-hour pain-free response was 43%. The likelihood of the headache recurring within 24 hours after getting pain relief was generally 30–40%. A lower dose (5 mg) is necessary if a patient is taking the beta blocker propranolol (Inderal). This medication is used to treat high blood pressure, angina, and anxiety, but also is one of the most commonly prescribed migraine preventive agents (see chapter 7). Side effects of rizatriptan are similar to those of sumatriptan and zolmitriptan.

Consistency studies have shown that about 80% of attacks over a year can be relieved by two hours with 10 mg tablets of rizatriptan in the people who choose to keep using the drug. This rate is similar to that for sumatriptan and zolmitriptan tablets.

Rizatriptan may be the fastest of the fast-acting triptan oral tablets. Several studies have been conducted to see if the fact that rizatriptan reaches maximal concentration in the blood faster than sumatriptan and zolmitriptan translates into a faster onset of action for a person trying to get rid of a migraine with rizatriptan than with the other two fast onset triptans. There is some controversy in the statistical analysis of these direct comparison studies, but the bottom line is that rizatriptan tablets may work slightly faster than sumatriptan and zolmitriptan tablets. Obviously, no tablet works as fast as a nasal spray or injection, since these two forms bypass the need for gastrointestinal absorption, which delays onset of action.

Almotriptan (Axert)

Approximately a quarter of a dose of almotriptan (Axert) is eliminated by the kidneys, but it also has liver elimination by different enzyme systems. The multiple ways that it gets out of the body reduces the chance of an interaction with other drugs, which is an advantage of this medication.

The likelihood of obtaining pain relief within two hours is around 60%, about the same as sumatriptan. In studies, almotriptan had milder nuisance side effects than the other fast acting triptans (except the 25 mg sumatriptan and 5 mg rizatriptan). The low side effects and the lack of interaction with other drugs make almotriptan an easy to use and effective oral medication.

Eletriptan (Relpax)

Eletriptan (Relpax) is broken down exclusively in the liver by the cytochrome P450 enzyme system, not by the MAO system. Certain antibiotics and anti-fungal/yeast medications that share the P450 enzyme breakdown route may interact with eletriptan. Competition for the enzyme system may lead to elevation of the eletriptan level in the blood when these medications are used together. The medications that should be avoided with eletriptan include the macrolide antibiotics such as erythromycin, clarithromycin (Biaxin), and the antifungal ketoconazole.

The likelihood of getting pain relief in two hours ranges from 54–65% with the recommended starting dose of 40 mg. The likelihood of the headache recurring within 24 hours after pain relief is achieved ranges from 19–31%, a fairly wide range in the various studies.

Eletriptan has been compared to sumatriptan in several studies. They are probably about equivalent in effectiveness.

This underscores the similarities of the Type I fast-acting oral triptans. The effectiveness of these medications is equivalent, although there are decided individual preferences. For greater speed, nasal sprays and the sumatriptan injection are clearly superior. For convenience, a melt works very well. For patients with variable migraine, the use of sumatriptan with three forms of dosing, or zolmitriptan with tablet, melt, and nasal spray will be optimal. Otherwise, when using oral tablets, the Type I triptans are more similar than they are different. The advent of the new rapid release sumatriptan tablets has not been fully evaluated at the time of this writing.

Triptan Group II
Naratriptan (Amerge)

Naratriptan (Amerge), a slow-acting triptan, has unique properties that are useful in treating migraine, despite providing relief with a slow onset of effect. Close to half of patients obtain headache relief within the first two hours, and 60–68% by four hours. In general, Group II triptans (naratriptan and frovatriptan) take twice as long as Group I triptans to provide relief. They should be used only in migraine coming on slowly, and are not optimal for migraine on awakening or galloping migraine. As with all triptans, speed of effect and overall efficacy can be maximized by taking the medication early in an attack, when pain is mild.

About 70% of naratriptan is eliminated by the kidneys. The rest is metabolized by the liver, but not by the MAO system.

If naratriptan is slower in effect than the fast-acting triptans and works in fewer people, why use it? The answer has to do with other properties of naratriptan.

First, it has few side effects at the doses used. Most studies have found side effects are similar to placebo. So naratriptan is a "gentle triptan," similar to almotriptan. It is great for people with tendency to experience side effects. It is important to remember, however, that the side effects patients experience with triptans are not related to the chance that the drug will narrow coronary arteries. So even though naratriptan and almotriptan are gentle, they still cannot be used in people with vascular or heart disease.

After taking naratriptan and achieving pain relief, the likelihood of the headache recurring within the first 24 hours is around 20%. This compares favorably with a recurrence rate of 30–40% for sumatriptan, zolmitriptan, and rizatriptan. If a patient gets frequent or multiple recurrence from the fast-acting triptans, naratriptan may be an excellent choice. Frequent recurrence means recurrence on most of the migraines treated. Multiple recurrence means more than one recurrence on the same migraine. With multiple recurrence the migraine never switches off—and the use of multiple doses of a triptan for days is expensive.

Multiple recurrence is particularly a problem with long migraines, such as those prolonged headaches occurring around menstruation. Naratriptan taken early in the attack has the potential to give relief without recurrence.

Some people will begin with a fast-acting triptan, especially if they wake up with a migraine, but then use naratriptan for the recurrence the next day. We do not know that this treatment results in a lower multiple recurrence rate after the first recurrence is treated with naratriptan, but it is well worth a try as long as different triptans are not mixed on the same day.

Interestingly, naratriptan has also been shown to be effective in preventing menstrual migraine. Naratriptan 1 mg tablets taken twice daily for a total of 5 days, beginning two days before the expected onset in those patients with regular menstrual migraine, prevented at least half of the menstrual attacks.

Naratriptan, when given to people who chose to use it over a year, resulted in pain relief in about 70% of attacks at 4 hours. So, its consistency is a bit lower than the fast acting triptans.

Naratriptan is sometimes referred to as "sumatriptan-lite, suma-triptan-long." It is sumatriptan-lite because it works in fewer people than sumatriptan, but has fewer side effects. It is sumatriptan-long because it takes longer to work than sumatriptan, but is more likely to give sustained relief without recurrence.

Frovatriptan (Frova)
Frovatriptan (Frova) is the other slow-onset, long-lasting triptan. It takes 25 hours for half of a frovatriptan dose to be eliminated from the body, four times as long lasting as naratriptan. Frovatriptan is half eliminated by the kidneys and half by the liver, but not by

Table 6.2 The Group II triptans				
Drug	Brand name	Form	Dose (mg)	Directions
Naratriptan	Amerge	Tablet	1, 2.5 (2.5 is recommended dose)	Can repeat in 4 h, maximum 5 mg/24 h
Frovatriptan	Frova	Tablet	2.5	Can repeat in 2 h, maximum 7.5 mg/24 h

the MAO system. Fewer people respond to frovatriptan than to Group I triptans.

About 41% of patients obtain pain relief from frovatriptan by two hours. Around 60% have a headache response by four hours. So, again similar to naratriptan, the four-hour numbers for frovatriptan look like the two-hour numbers for the fast-acting triptans. Interestingly, when frovatriptan was given to patients over a year, there was a subset of people for whom the frovatriptan worked reliably within two hours.

The likelihood of the migraine returning was low with frovatriptan, ranging from 7–25%.

Patients who had a faster onset of action with frovatriptan when they used it over a year had a very low likelihood, about 6%, of their migraine returning within 24 hours of obtaining pain relief. So not only is there clearly a subset of people who will get reasonably fast action from frovatriptan, they are the same people who have a very low likelihood of migraine recurrence with frovatriptan. Reported side effects are similar to the other triptans. Therefore, frovatriptan may be optimal for long headaches, such as some menstrual migraines. Frovatriptan was recently found to prevent menstrual migraine when taken before onset of the attack and daily through menses, similar to naraptriptan.

Rescue Therapy

The oral triptans work on 80–95% of attacks, depending on the drug, and injectable sumatriptan on up to 90% of attacks. For the remaining few attacks when these medications fail, patients need a backup plan—called "rescue therapy" to distinguish it from the migraine-specific medication that usually will restore normal function. Rescue means pain relief, usually nausea relief, but sleep will often get rid of a migraine when nothing else does. This may be due to the outpouring of serotonin that occurs during sleep, or due to inhibition of the migraine central generator during sleep.

Opioid or Narcotic Rescue

For pain relief, narcotic or opioid therapy is often recommended. However, there are serious warnings to keep in mind before using this treatment, and for this reason I always recommend trying injectable sumatriptan first.

Narcotic use must be very infrequent. I prefer that my patients use rescue therapy no more than twice monthly. And to safely use narcotics there must be no previous history of drug or alcohol abuse; otherwise, there will be significant addiction risk.

Even without a history of alcoholism or drug abuse, if migraines and consequent opioid rescue are frequent, the risk is quite high of transforming from occasional migraines to daily headache or rebound from the opioids. And that can occur with as few as three doses of oral or one dose of non-oral narcotic pain medication per week.

When rescue pain medication is needed, the patient is usually at the vomiting or severely nauseated stage of a migraine. At that point, oral narcotics rarely work, often worsen nausea, and most of the time are inadequately absorbed due to gastric stasis or vomiting.

Non-oral alternatives include rectal suppositories of hydro-morphone (Dilaudid), nasal butorphanol (Stadol), or injectable narcotics such as meperidine (Demerol). The hydromorphone is easy to use and rarely causes side effects, but some patients find it too mild to put them to sleep.

On the other hand, nasal butorphanol obeys what is called, in headache circles, the "rule of halves." About half of the people who try nasal butorphanol hate it, because it can cause odd side effects, such as intense, unpleasant feelings up to and including hallucinations.

Of the remaining half of patients who use it, half like nasal butorphanol too much. They run a serious risk of addiction. I have never been able to detoxify a patient from overuse of nasal butorphanol out of the hospital, because the craving is so great.

That leaves the patients for whom it fits nicely for rescue. Under those circumstances, nasal butorphanol gives good pain relief with sedation (one sniff is like one shot of narcotic). And it bypasses the gastrointestinal tract.

Occasionally, a trip to an emergency room or doctor's office is necessary for injection. Injection rescue should be limited to no more than once a month, and any trip of this sort suggests the need to improve preventive treatment at home.

Antinausea Medications

Most patients require an antinausea medication for rescue. Once again, oral medications are rarely tolerated so rectal suppositories are often used, including prochlorperazine (Compazine), promethazine (Phenergan), and trimethobenzamide (Tigan).

7. Preventing Migraines

Non-medication Prevention

Trigger Reduction

There are a number of steps that can be taken to prevent migraine that do not require medication. One is trigger reduction.

The concept of trigger reduction is that, if migraine is caused by a hyperexcitable brain, exposure to certain external factors can set off a firing of the nerves in the brain that cause migraine. These triggers do not cause headache in a person without migraine, but they commonly trigger migraine in those susceptible. In fact, some headache specialists think that migraine should be diagnosed by the fact that it can be triggered by recognizable triggers that often do not cause other types of headaches or neurologic illnesses. This is recognizing migraine by the company that it keeps.

Trigger reduction is useful in reducing the frequency of migraine, but it rarely completely eliminates migraine. Triggers are sometimes unreliable and do not cause migraine with each exposure, and even after elimination of known triggers, it often happens that migraines still occur.

Common triggers are shown in table 7.1. Before embarking on a discovery search, I strongly recommend that a patient find a medication that will reliably stop migraine attacks. The patient can then experiment with a potential trigger, and if a migraine is precipitated, it can be stopped reliably with the medication to avoid disability. If the trigger reproducibly brings on a migraine, it is clearly worth eliminating. Doing so will reduce the frequency of migraines and add control over some of the attacks.

Keeping a headache diary or calendar is the best tool in discovering triggers (see chapter 5 and table 7.1).

Table 7.1 Triggers of migraine
Foods
Nitrates and prepared meats
*Alcohol and red wine
*Cheese, especially strong cheddar cheese, Gruyere, Brie, Camembert
Certain fruits such as citrus and pineapple
Bananas
*Monosodium glutamate (MSG)
*Aspartame (Nutrasweet)
Dairy products
Canned eggs
Nuts, peanut butter
Onions
Yogurt, sour cream
Avocado
Herring (fermented, pickled, marinated foods)
Chicken livers
Cured meats (bologna, salami, pepperoni, hot dogs, bacon)
Other triggers
Fasting, skipping a meal
Menstruation and ovulation, alterations in sex hormones
Exercise and exertion
Sexual activity
Medications, such as oral contraceptive pills
*Stress and let-down from stress
*Weather change
Video display terminals, TV, and movies
Jet lag

(continued)

Table 7.1 (*continued*)
High altitude
Plane rides
Odors and exposure to cigarette smoke, fumes, perfume
Light, including sunlight and fluorescent light
*Changes in sleep, such as sleeping late or fatigue
* Most common

Caffeine, the Double-edged Sword

Taken occasionally, caffeine can actually help get rid of a migraine. Caffeine is added to many acute treatments for migraine, and seems to improve the effectiveness of these medications, although the mechanism for the synergism is unknown. Caffeine is added to aspirin (Anacin), aspirin and acetaminophen (Excedrin), butalbital and other over-the-counter analgesics (Fiorinal), and ergotamine (Cafergot).

However, when consumed daily, caffeine is less likely to be helpful in getting rid of an acute attack. If a person uses 100–200 mg on a daily basis (one cup of coffee can have 100 mg or more of caffeine, and a can of soda can have 40 mg), the wearing off of the caffeine can cause headache. This is another rebound headache (see chapter 8). Tapering down or off of caffeine can be very useful in reducing the frequency of headache.

Life-style

Life-style changes can reduce the frequency of migraines, and are non-pharmacologic, active interventions well suited for prevention.

It seems a deceptively simple observation: keeping regular living habits can be extremely important in keeping the headaches down. The opposite is what most migraine people notice—that if they miss sleep or miss meals, they pay the price in a migraine.

My patients tell me that merely deciding to go to bed and wake at somewhat fixed times helps eliminate quite a few headaches per year, and sometimes per month. I sometimes intercede with employers on behalf of my patients with migraine to establish a work schedule that does not involve switching shifts.

If a patient knows that skipping a meal triggers attacks, or that eating seems to stave off migraine, why not try regular meals? When explained to families, life-style changes are often simple interventions from which everyone will benefit by fewer migraines. Please see the headache diary in chapter 5, table 5.1.

We all know that stress can trigger attacks, and in fact, stress is the most common trigger of migraines. Relaxation can help prevent attacks, and many psychologists can provide relaxation tapes and exercises to keep stress down. But, more than that, if a certain stressful situation triggers attacks, a patient can enlist friends, fellow employees, boss, and family to help avoid them.

Some people get migraine from "letdown" after stress, at least as many as those who get migraine at the peak of stress. Letdown migraine can happen on weekends after a stressful week of work.

Even worse is what I call "Maui migraine," when a person works hard to get on vacation and has the first three days of the holiday ruined by a migraine attack. This form of migraine is very difficult to prevent and sometimes requires one of the "mini-prevention" medications described at the end of this chapter.

For those who have migraine from peak of stress, I always recommend regular aerobic exercise as the first step in stress reduction. If a patient can obtain relaxation tapes and exercises, they are easy to use and not too time consuming.

The next step up the ladder for reduction of stress is learning biofeedback or meditation. Biofeedback is a technique that teaches awareness and control of certain key activities related to muscles and blood vessels. Training can result in enhanced control of these functions, which then leads to a feeling of well-being and reduction of stress.

Some headache specialists feel that people who are very tense, and in whom tense muscles can be documented, are particularly good candidates for biofeedback. However, the technique can be time consuming.

Meditation is also called the "relaxation response." Transcendental meditation involves picking a "mantra" or word to repeat. Meditation, like biofeedback, takes practice, and with time results in a sort of self-hypnotic trance, which is very relaxing. Repetitive relaxation reduces the frequency and severity of migraine.

Physical Therapy

Physical therapy and massage can sometimes help with tense muscles. As noted before, when the central generator for migraine is activated, it turns on adjacent nuclei in the lower brainstem and neck that cause pain and muscle spasm during the attack. This is one of the reasons for neck pain in migraine. Physical therapy and massage (passive therapies) have not been documented to reduce migraine frequency as much as regular aerobic exercise or relaxation techniques (active therapies), but can reduce muscle tension, which some people find helpful.

Alternative Care

Patients are continually being bombarded by proposed alternative therapies. Magnets, chiropractic, osteopathy, naturopathy, homeopathy, herbs, unusual physical treatments like rolfing and shiatsu—it seems every week brings a new claim. There is usually little legitimate evidence to support them. The only way to determine if a treatment is effective is the double-blind, placebo-controlled, randomized scientific study, in which similar patients are given what appears to be the same treatment for the same disease, but one of the treatments is placebo. Neither patients nor doctors know which is placebo until after the treatment is administered and data are collected.

Faith, or the placebo effect, can make any treatment work, including an alternative one, for up to three months or more, although why this power of suggestion is so strong is unknown. However, after about three months reality begins to re-assert itself, and the full impact of the disease and the lack of effectiveness of a treatment begin to show. So, to determine if a treatment works, it needs to be compared with placebo, to see how much more effective it is than the placebo.

Sometimes the results are surprising. I used an anti-depressant medication to prevent migraines on many patients with what I thought was great success. Two double-blind, placebo-controlled studies then showed this medication utterly ineffective in migraine prevention when compared to placebo. I was either seeing very rare, individual patient responses, or a placebo response propelled by the wish that my patients and I had to make the drug work.

But it helps to keep an open mind. A preliminary placebo-controlled study suggested that botulinum injections in the head and neck may prevent migraine in some people. Multiple further studies on botulinum toxin injections appear to confirm an effectiveness similar to other conventional preventive therapies. Who could have conceived of this treatment being effective, since no mechanism for its effectiveness had even been suggested until it was tried?

On the other hand, two European double-blind studies have found multiple naturopathic treatments of herbs and chemicals for migraine prevention no more effective than placebo, so I am inclined to think that that avenue holds little promise.

Vitamin, herb, and mineral supplements have been found to be helpful in some scientific studies, specifically vitamin B2, feverfew, and magnesium. A few thoughts on these treatments: First, if a treatment is working beyond three months, and not harmful, stay with it. Second, many ideas and remedies that close-minded and dogmatic people dismiss turn out to be effective in scientific study. The key is to demand scientific study.

Finally, it is worth remembering that in the 1994 Dietary Supplement Health and Education Act, Congress classified herbal medicines as supplements, not drugs, and therefore not subject to FDA regulation. Their contents are unmonitored and unevaluated, as are their claims. Scientific study is not required for their marketing. So, as a doctor, I often have no information with which to help my patients decide on the safety or effectiveness of various herbs, health foods, and naturopathic and homeopathic remedies.

Preventive Medication for Migraine

The decision to take daily medication to prevent migraine is one of the most difficult decisions a migraine patient has to make. The purpose of taking daily preventive medication is to reduce the frequency, severity, and/or duration of migraine attacks. Generally, effective prevention also improves the response to the acute abortive medications that take away the migraines that break through.

It is important to realize that most preventive medication does not eliminate all migraine attacks. I tell my patients that if the daily medication reduces the frequency of the attacks by 50%, they are doing very well. That is the goal I set for daily preventive medication.

Why would a patient take daily preventive medication? If the frequency of migraines is high, reducing how often migraines occur looks attractive, even if there are reliable medications to abort the headaches.

How many migraines a month would it take to warrant prevention with daily medication? The answer should be individualized, not decreed by a physician or insurance plan.

It is sometimes stated that people with more than two or three attacks per month should always be given daily preventive medication. I am more flexible. If one of my patients has one to two migraines per week, aborts them reliably and easily with a triptan, and wants to avoid daily drugs, I do not push the issue. I do bring up the option of daily prevention in people with frequent headaches.

However, there are other reasons to consider daily drugs for migraine. If a person is missing work or time at home—that is, experiencing a lot of disability due to the migraines—then intervening to reduce the frequency of the attacks can be economical, or can help socially. The cost of daily medication must be balanced against the cost of acute medication and the cost of the work loss. One trip to the ER can drive up the cost for treatment enormously.

If a patient has not found acceptable acute medications that reliably terminate migraine attacks, or if other health issues preclude using the major anti-migraine medications, prevention becomes a more reasonable choice. With the presence of heart disease (contraindicating the use of triptans or ergots) or ulcer disease (preventing the use of certain anti-inflammatory drugs), it becomes quite difficult to stop a headache, and prevention may be the better option.

Even when the acute drugs work, the side effects may sometimes be unacceptable, and so prevention is chosen. And the character of attacks may lead to the decision to go on preventive drugs. I have had patients who hate their attacks so much that they want to avoid even a single migraine per month, even when they have good abortive medication. In that setting, prevention is reasonable.

Sometimes I strongly recommend daily preventive medication. This occurs when I worry that the characteristics of the migraine may be dangerous to a person's health. If the migraine is accompanied by severe weakness of one side of the body, if an aura goes on for hours, or if there are other complicated neurologic symptoms with an attack, I may recommend daily preventive treatment to minimize the frequency of the attacks, or to minimize the likelihood of stroke associated with the migraines.

The trick with the daily preventive medication is to use the lowest dose possible. I will sometimes put one drug on at a low or moderate dose; if it does not work, I will then add another. This is called *co-pharmacy*. When one adds in this way, the whole can sometimes be greater than the sum of the parts.

Another approach is to increase one medicine dose until it either stops the headaches or the dose is so high that it causes side effects, then lower it slightly. I generally do not use this approach because it means giving the patient side effects, and the other approach of adding the second medicine when the first is still at a moderate dose works well. It sometimes takes up to three months for a preventive medication to work, so patience is critical. Completely eliminating the migraines often involves increasing the dose too high to be tolerated.

What evidence do we have that preventive medication works? The FDA periodically reviews applications in which a pharmaceutical company presents data suggesting that their certain drug should be approved for preventive treatment of migraine. When the FDA approves a medication for this purpose, it means the evidence is strong.

The FDA has approved only four preventive treatments for migraine: propranolol (Inderal), timolol (Blocadren), divalproex sodium (Depakote), and methysergide (Sansert). A fifth medication, topiramate (Topamax), may be approved in 2003. This does not mean that no other drugs work, of course.

There are medications for which the evidence is strong for prevention, but where the drug company has never submitted an FDA application. Recently, an arm of the government, the American Health Care Policy and Research (AHCPR), has reviewed all the evidence on all the preventive medications and graded the drugs, placing them into groups of effectiveness (see table 7.2).

Group 1 consists of medications of medium to high effectiveness, with strong evidence for their effectiveness and mild to moderate side effects. Evidence was less strong for medications in Group 2.

Group 3 was divided into two parts. Group 3a drugs were felt to be effective based on clinical experience, but there was no statistical evidence of effectiveness, and Group 3b medications had significant side effects. Group 4 medications showed medium to high effectiveness, good strength of evidence, but with side effect concerns. Group 5 drugs were felt to be ineffective in migraine prevention.

Group 1 Medications: Strong Evidence for Effectiveness

Beta blockers

Beta blockers are medications that block some effects of adrenaline. They lower blood pressure, slow heart rate, and have other cardiovascular effects and so are often prescribed by cardiologists and internists for a variety of ailments, including high blood pressure and angina; they are the standard of care for treatment post-heart attacks.

They also reduce anxiety and "steady the nerves." Musicians will sometimes take a short acting beta blocker before performing.

Table 7.2 Major U.S. preventive medications for migraine as graded by the American Health Care Policy and Research Committee

Group 1

Amitriptyline, divalproex sodium, propranolol, timolol

Group 2

Aspirin, atenolol, fenoprofen, feverfew, flurbiprofen, fluoxetine, gabapentin, ketoprofen, magnesium, mefanamic acid, metoprolol, nadolol, naproxen with and without sodium, nimodipine, verapamil, vitamin B2 (riboflavin)

Group 3a

Cyproheptadine, buproprion, diltiazem, doxepin, fluvoxamine, ibuprofen, imipramine, mirtazepine, nortriptyline, paroxetine, protriptyline, sertraline, tiagabine, topiramate, trazodone, venlafaxine

Group 3b

Methylergonovine, phenelzine

Group 4

Methysergide

Group 5

Carbamazepine, clonidine, indomethacin, lamotrigine

Beta blockers that are effective in migraine include propranolol (Inderal) and timolol (Blocadren), both of which are approved for prevention of migraine by the FDA and both of which are in Group 1. Other beta blockers that work well in migraine prevention include atenolol (Tenormin), metoprolol (Lopressor, Toprol), and nadolol (Corgard), all of which are in Group 2.

Beta blockers can cause drowsiness, or more frequently sluggishness or a lack of energy. Even more importantly, they can precipitate depression, especially in people with a history of depression. These

Drug	Brand name	Doses (mg)	Instructions for use in migraine
Propranolol	Inderal	60–160	Slow increase, long acting (LA), easier to use
Nadolol	Corgard	40–160	Slow increase
Metoprolol	Lopressor, Toprol	50–100	Slow increase
Atenolol	Tenormin	50–100	Slow increase
Timolol	Blocadren	10–20	Slow increase

Table 7.3 Beta blockers used in migraine

medications can also disturb sleep, and occasionally cause erectile dysfunction.

As stated above, beta blockers have many cardiovascular effects, so not everyone can take them. They lower the blood pressure and pulse. They can interfere with regular aerobic athletics, because heart rate will stay slow. They should not be used in people with congestive heart failure. Beta blockers can make asthma worse, usually in people with a history of asthma. And they exacerbate Raynaud's phenomenon (see chapter 6, section on ergotamine tartrate). Beta blockers should not be used by diabetics.

However, for the most part beta blockers are well tolerated, and sometimes the multiple effects of the drug can help treat two health problems at once. This is referred to as treating co-morbidity.

For example, if a patient has hypertension and frequent migraine, a beta blocker will take care of both at once. Beta blockers can reduce stage fright, so a performer with this and migraine will want a beta blocker. With angina or heart disease, a physician will likely recommend a beta blocker anyway.

Another example is anxiety or panic with migraine. Beta blockers can reduce anxiety and "the jitters" and lower the frequency of the migraines with one medication. Propranolol is generally prescribed for this situation.

Doses of beta blockers that suppress migraine are variable, and sometimes low doses work well. Recommended doses are shown in table 7.3.

Beta blockers block one type of adrenalin receptors, the beta type, by binding to them. There may be an adrenalin-activated pathway that turns on the excitatory serotonin receptors, the 5-HT$_2$ receptors. When the 5-HT$_2$ receptors are activated, migraine may be activated. So perhaps beta blockers prevent the activation of the 5-HT$_2$ excitatory system by adrenalin, and therefore prevent activation of migraine itself.

Divalproex sodium (Depakote)

Divalproex sodium is another effective Group 1 migraine prevention drug. The ingredients of this medication have been used in the treatment of epilepsy since the 1960s in the United Kingdom and since the 1970s in the U.S.

Divalproex is probably nearly as effective as the beta blockers in preventing migraine, but unlike the beta blockers it has no effect on the heart or blood pressure. The advantage for divalproex is clearly for people who cannot take beta blockers. Divalproex does not interfere with aerobic exercise.

Two groups of people with migraine can particularly benefit from divalproex, because they have other illnesses that divalproex can help besides migraine.

The first group is patients with both epilepsy and migraine; divalproex works to prevent most kinds of epilepsy, although at doses higher than are needed to treat migraine.

Divalproex can also be used to stabilize the mood of people with manic depressive illness (bipolar disorder). It is approved by the FDA for this use as well, and is similar to lithium in its mood-stabilizing effect. So for people with both bipolar disorder and migraine, divalproex is an excellent choice.

The disadvantage of divalproex is its potential for side effects. At high dose, the list of side effects it can cause can be quite alarming: hair loss, drowsiness, tremor, nausea, diarrhea, weight gain, foot swelling, and inflammation of the liver, pancreas, or bone marrow. At low doses, it tends not to give these side effects, but if it does cause any of them, divalproex should not be used.

The FDA suggests beginning with a low dose, 250 mg twice daily, or 500 mg of the extended release form (ER) and many headache specialists begin patients at an even lower dose, such as 125 mg twice daily and move the dose up only if the patient needs a higher dose. I rarely treat with doses higher than 1000 mg/day because I do not want my patients to get the side effects.

What I tell my patients is that taking divalproex is a gamble. The gamble is that they get a 50% reduction in the migraine frequency at a dose low enough not to give them side effects. If it does not work at doses that do not give side effects, they should not take it. Only if the dose used is tolerated do I think it a good idea to stay on it.

There has long been concern about the potential of divalproex to cause liver problems. This can be a big problem in children; in adults, it probably causes liver problems only when combined with another medication, such as phenobarbital, other barbiturates such as butalbital, or tranquilizers.

Before a patient goes on divalproex alone, I check blood work including blood count, liver, and pancreas tests one time before starting the drug, to establish no problem at baseline. I then recheck the bloods at the next visit after the person has been on the divalproex. For a patient who is going to be on divalproex and other drugs at the same time, I generally check bloods at least yearly.

Divalproex can also cause significant birth defects, so I require fertile female patients on divalproex to be on birth control pills or have a failsafe contraceptive method.

How does divalproex work? It may have several ways of turning off migraine.

First, it may work inside the brain by inhibiting some of the excitatory activity associated with migraine. It may increase the effect of gamma-amino butyric acid (GABA), an inhibitory neurotransmitter, or it may work via a serotonin mechanism.

The GABA inhibitory effect of divalproex has been shown to turn off the inflammation that occurs in the meninges during migraine. Central nervous system action may inhibit the central generator of migraine, while the peripheral effect in the meninges may deactivate one of the mechanisms for pain in migraine, namely the inflammation. Increasing GABA effect may also reduce the overall hyperexcitability of the nerves in the migraine-susceptible brain. Possibly because of its multiple modes of action, divalproex has become one of the mainstays of migraine prevention.

Tricyclics

Tricyclics are versatile medications originally developed as antidepressants. Amitriptyline (Elavil) is highly effective in migraine treatment. Amitriptyline breaks down in the body to nortriptyline (Pamelor), and nortriptyline is often prescribed in preference to amitriptyline, because it has less intense side effects. Other effective tricyclics include doxepin (Sinequan), protriptyline (Vivactil), and, probably, imipramine (Tofranil), all of which are in Group 3a with nortriptyline.

Although highly effective with migraine, the limiting problems when using tricyclics are the side effects. The tricyclics can cause what I tell my patients are the "four horsemen of the apocalypse," namely dry mouth, constipation, sedation, and weight gain. They can also seriously worsen glaucoma and can aggravate prostate problems. Many of the side effects are derived from the fact that tricyclics block the neurotransmitter acetylcholine (they have anti-cholinergic effects). Unfortunately, blocking acetylcholine does not help prevent migraine, so the side effects are just unneeded baggage for these medications.

Side effects are mildest with nortriptyline and protriptyline, but unfortunately are greatest with amitriptyline, for which there is the strongest evidence of effectiveness. By using the lowest doses, by taking the drug at night like a sleeping pill, and by preferring nortriptyline, the side effects can be minimized.

There is some evidence that tricyclics can cause abnormal cardiac rhythms in people with heart disease. Many doctors will not prescribe them for patients with heart disease, and will instead choose a migraine preventive medication with no likelihood of causing a cardiac problem, such as an anti-epilepsy drug.

Table 7.4 Tricyclics used in migraine				
Drug	**Brand name**	**Doses (mg)**	**Directions**	**Concern**
Amitriptyline	Elavil	10–150	Slow increase	Dry mouth, glaucoma, constipation, sedation, weight gain
Nortriptyline	Pamelor	Same as above	Same as above	Same as above
Doxepin	Sinequan	Same as above	Same as above	Same as above
Imipramine	Tofranil	Same as above	Same as above	Same as above
Protriptyline	Vivactil	5–10	Take in AM	Activation, insomnia, glaucoma, constipation

Because tricyclics (with the exception of protriptyline) do cause sleepiness, they are often the perfect non-habit-forming sleeping pill. Thus two problems can be solved with one medication.

Tricyclics are effective anti-pain medications, and unlike triptans they work on almost all types of pain, in addition to headache. Tricyclics reduce neck pain, back pain, pain from shingles, and other types of nerve pain. So people with several types of pain, sleep disturbance, and frequent migraines can really benefit from taking a nightly tricyclic. And the tricyclics are powerful antidepressants.

How do tricyclics work? They appear to make serotonin and adrenaline more available at the right receptor sites, for example

5-HT$_1$ inhibitory receptors. They block the reuptake of these neurotransmitters after release, like the selective serotonin reuptake inhibitors. And they slowly reduce the number of excitatory serotonin 5-HT$_2$ receptors, so that there is less chance to activate migraine. They also probably suppress the migraine central generator.

Recommended doses for the tricyclics are given in table 7.4.

Group 2 Medications

Calcium channel blockers

Calcium channel blockers work in fewer people than the Group 1 medications, but are often prescribed because of their fewer side effects. Some people should be prescribed calcium channel blockers as their first migraine preventive medication.

There has been a resurgence of interest in the use of calcium channel blockers because of a recent advance in genetics (see chapter 9). It was discovered that familial hemiplegic migraine (FHM) patients often have an abnormal gene that codes for an abnormal calcium ion channel. Calcium channel blockers block the abnormal calcium gate in these patients, stopping virtually all of their migraines and the auras and paralysis as well.

Naturally, this has led to the question of whether more common forms of migraine have a similar basis. And if they do, will calcium channel blockers help prevent those migraine types?

Some headache specialists feel that there is a greater likelihood that calcium channel blockers will prevent migraine in people with migraine with aura. The idea is that all aura is similar, including the usual forms as well as the aura in FHM, and all is caused by cortical spreading depression (see chapter 4). Recent data also suggest subtle abnormalities in those portions of the brain with the highest calcium channel concentrations in patients with aura.

I have had good success in using calcium channel blockers in my patients with migraine with aura, and the side effects are usually less than with Group 1 drugs. About 30% of patients will obtain at least a 50% reduction in their migraine frequency.

The calcium channel blocker available in the U.S. with the best evidence for effectiveness is verapamil (Calan, Isoptin, Verelan, Covera), which is in Group 2. I usually begin with this drug if the side-effect profile permits.

Verapamil and other calcium channel blockers have significant cardiovascular effects that can limit their use. They lower blood pressure and can alter cardiac rhythm. Certain cardiac conditions preclude their use, and if the patient is starting with low blood pressure to begin with, he or she may not tolerate this form of medication.

Occasionally, calcium channel blockers will trigger a potentially dangerous heart rhythm or palpitations. I warn people to call immediately if they get those rare palpitations.

Unlike beta blockers, calcium channel blockers usually do not cause exercise intolerance. Although they lower blood pressure, they rarely lower pulse, and this allows most people to exercise normally— a distinct advantage.

All the calcium channel blockers can cause foot swelling. This is usually less of a problem with verapamil than with some of the others. Verapamil, on the other hand, can cause severe constipation, so I always ask my patients if they have a tendency to constipation. If they do, verapamil is not for them. The mechanism for these side effects is not clear.

What about the side effect profile makes using verapamil so attractive? It is what verapamil usually does not do. It usually does not cause drowsiness, weight gain, or cognitive fuzziness, unlike what can happen with any of the Group 1 drugs. Verapamil also usually does not cause weight gain, dry mouth, or tremor, as it does not have anticholinergic effects.

If a patient has a history of constipation, then I try a calcium channel blocker that does not generally cause constipation, such as amlodipine (Norvasc). Many specialists have found it very helpful, but larger studies need to be done.

The main problem with amlodipine is that it can cause foot swelling. If this occurs I usually try a mixture of amlodipine and benazepril called Lotrel. The benazepril can get rid of the foot

Table 7.5 Calcium channel blockers used in migraine				
Drug	Brand name	Dose (mg)	Directions	Concerns
Verapamil	Calan, Isoptin, Verelan, Covera	80–480	Short acting, three times daily; long acting, once or twice daily	Constipation, cardiac dysfunction, foot swelling
Diltiazem	Cardizem, Tiazec, Dilacor	90–300	Same as above	Same as above
Amlodipine	Norvasc	5–10	Get used to 5 before moving to 10	Foot swelling is main problem: if so, try Lotrel; also cardiac dysfunction
Nisoldipine	Sular	10–40	Twice daily	Cardiac dysfunction, foot swelling

swelling, allowing for the use of the amlodipine. Lotrel will some-times cause a cough; if it does, it is contraindicated.

There have been some reports that diltiazem (Cardizem, Tiazec, Dilacor) can help prevent migraine, although it too can cause constipation and foot swelling. Because of a lack of evidence of effectiveness, it is in Group 3a.

Nisoldipine (Sular) is less expensive than amlodipine. If it works and does not cause foot swelling, it saves some money. It has not been tested much in headache prevention and has not been grouped.

Nimodipine is used in some other countries, but in this country it is too expensive to be taken daily. Flunarazine (Sibelium) is perhaps the most effective migraine preventing calcium channel blocker, although it is not available in the U.S. It is available in Canada, Mexico, and Europe. Unfortunately, flunarazine can cause weight gain and depression, so its use can be limited. In Europe there is an attempt going forward to develop a calcium channel blocker as effective as flunarazine but without the side effects.

Nonsteroidal anti-inflammatory drugs

Nonsteroidal anti-inflammatory drugs (NSAIDs) taken daily can prevent migraine. Many of them are in Group 2, including fenoprofen (Nalfon), flurbiprofen (Ansaid), ketoprofen (Orudis, Oruvail), mefanamic acid (Ponstel), naproxen (Naprosyn), and naproxen sodium (Anaprox, Aleve, Naprelan). Ibuprofen (Advil, Motrin), which people report sometimes works, is in Group 3a.

NSAIDs block prostaglandin synthesis via cyclo-oxygenase (COX). There are two major cyclo-oxygenases—COX-1 and COX-2. COX-1 has important functions in the stomach, kidney, and platelets, while COX-2 is associated with inflammation. The older NSAIDs block both, preventing inflammation mediated by prostaglandins, but also setting up potential for adverse events in the stomach, kidneys, and platelets. If part of the mechanism of migraine pain is inflammation around the blood vessels of the meninges (see chapter 4), taking a chronic anti-inflammatory may prevent the inflammation from developing.

The problem with taking the older "two-pathway blocking" NSAIDs is their potential for side effects such as elevated blood pressure, heartburn and indigestion, gastroesophageal reflux disease (GERD), stomach ulcers, excess bleeding, and kidney disease. Some NSAIDs have a particularly high risk for producing ulcers, specifically ketorolac (Toradol), and the development of ulcers can be without symptoms until the ulcer bleeds.

Some doctors attempt to prevent stomach ulcers by simultaneously prescribing a proton pump inhibitor stomach-protecting medication—omeprazole [Prilosec] is the most widely used—or the histamine H2 blocker mild stomach protectors also available over the counter, such as ranitidine (Zantac), cimetidine

(Tagamet), famotidine (Pepcid), and nizatidine (Axid), all of which work by interfering with the stomach's ability to produce acid.

The risk of kidney dysfunction in people taking daily NSAIDs merits renal monitoring. Because most NSAIDs inhibit platelet function, increasing the risk for bleeding, their use must be discontinued before surgery.

The last major problem in taking daily NSAIDs is that the anti-inflammatories can actually cause daily headache via the habituation and rebound phenomenon (see chapter 8). In that situation, not only do they not work in preventing migraine, they can transform occasional migraine into chronic daily headache. Because of the potential for gastrointestinal problems, kidney problems, and rebound daily headache, some headache specialists recommend against using NSAIDs at all as daily preventive medications.

There are many groups of NSAIDs, and little evidence favoring one group or particular NSAID over another in the prevention of migraine. Conventionally, we tend to use the NSAIDs from Group 2 first; most headache specialists use naproxen or naproxen sodium first, although indomethacin (which is in Group 5), ketoprofen, and flurbiprofen are often used as well.

All anti-inflammatories inhibit cyclo-oxygenase, but the COX-2 inhibitors inhibit only those associated with inflammation. The three available at the time of this writing are celecoxib (Celebrex), rofecoxib (Vioxx), and valdecoxib (Bextra). The advantage of COX-2 inhibitors is that, because they do not usually cause ulcers or gastrointestinal upset, they can be used with greater safety.

Aspirin is the granddaddy of all nonsteroidal anti-inflammatories, and carries with it the same risks of daily use. Scientific studies have shown it to be effective in preventing migraine, but there is no agreement what dose will prevent migraine.

There is agreement that, if daily aspirin to prevent migraine is going to be tried, aspirin should be taken alone and not mixed with caffeine (Anacin) or caffeine plus acetaminophen (Excedrin). Those combination drugs should be used to get rid of a mild, non-disabling migraine, not to prevent migraine on a daily basis.

Table 7.6 The major NSAIDs used in migraine

Drug [non-aspirin NSAIDs]	Brand name	Form	Dose (mg)	Directions	Concerns
Ibuprofen	Advil, Motrin, Nuprin	Tablet	200 over the counter 400, 600, 800	1–3 times/day	Gastrointestinal ulcer, GERD Kidney, blood pressure
Naproxen (with or without sodium)	Without sodium: Naprosyn With sodium: Aleve, Anaprox, Naprelan	Tablet	220 over the counter 250, 375, 550 short acting 375, 500 long acting (Naprelan)	2–3 times/day short acting 1–2/day long acting (Naprelan)	Same as above
Fenoprofen	Nalfon	Tablet	200, 300, 600	2–3 times/day	Same as above
Flurbiprofen	Ansaid	Tablet	50, 100	2–3 times/day	Same as above
Ketoprofen	Orudis, Oruvail	Tablet	25 over the counter 50, 75 short acting 200 long acting (Oruvail)	2–3 times/day, short acting 1 time/day long acting (Oruvail)	Same as above

Indomethacin	Indocin	Capsule, suppository, syrup	25, 50 short acting	3 times/day, short acting	Gastrointestinal ulcer, GERD
			75 long acting 50 suppository	2 times/day, long acting	Mental changes Eye problems Kidney, blood pressure
Mefanamic acid	Ponstel	Capsule	250	2–3 times/day	Gastrointestinal ulcer, GERD Kidney, blood pressure
Meclofenamate	Meclomen	Tablet	50–100	2 times/day	Same as above
Ketorolac	Toradol	Tablet, injection	10 tablet	2–3 times/day, orally	Same as above, but the ulcer risk is much higher and the
			15, 30, 60 injection	intramuscular or intravenous injections can also be given	number of uses per week should be severely limited
[COX-2 Inhibitors]					
Celecoxib	Celebrex	Tablet	100, 200	Once daily	Ulcer risk is lower
Rofecoxib	Vioxx	Tablet	12.5, 25, 50	1–2 times daily	Ulcer risk is lower
Valdecoxib	Bextra	Tablet	10, 20	Once daily	Ulcer risk is lower

Some studies suggest taking a regular aspirin daily (300–325 mg), others one every other day. Another suggestion is to take a "baby aspirin" (81 mg) daily.

These doses are low enough that they will not usually cause rebound or daily headache to develop. However, it may take several months for the aspirin to reduce the frequency of migraines—if it has any effect at all.

Gabapentin (Neurontin)

Gabapentin (Neurontin), another antiseizure medication, is in Group 2. Gabapentin reduces migraine frequency by 50% or more in at least a third of patients who take it at the proper dose. No one knows how gabapentin works, but like divalproex, it may inhibit the central generator for migraine.

Gabapentin is a safe medication, but less likely to be effective than Group 1 drugs. It only rarely causes weight gain, unlike divalproex and tricyclics. But it has some drawbacks as well. It is very expensive at the doses found to prevent migraine. And because gabapentin is short acting, it needs to be taken three times daily, which is inconvenient.

The biggest problems with gabapentin are the side effects of drowsiness and dizziness. These are common enough that I often begin by prescribing the lowest dose and raise the amount very slowly, beginning with a pediatric dose, 100 mg, taken at night. The lowest dose that worked in the big study was 1800 mg/day, though some people do respond to lower doses; the highest recommended dose is 4800 mg/day.

A number of opportunities exist to treat co-morbidities with gabapentin. There is some evidence that gabapentin can stabilize mood in people with manic depressive illness, similar to divalproex and lithium. It is a very reasonable choice for people with bipolar illness who want to prevent migraine.

Gabapentin is a powerful anti-pain medication. Like amitriptyline, it can reduce the pain from the neck, back, or nerves in the rest of the body. And it can treat body pain at much lower doses than are necessary to prevent migraine. Gabapentin was initially approved by the FDA as an anti-epilepsy drug, so people with epilepsy and migraine can use it to treat both illnesses.

Riboflavin (vitamin B2), magnesium, and feverfew

Patients frequently ask if there is any "more natural" way to prevent migraine than prescription medications. They are interested in vitamin therapy, mineral supplements, and herbs for treatment.

Whenever they ask, I talk to them about three options: riboflavin (vitamin B2), magnesium, and feverfew. The evidence of effectiveness is strongest for riboflavin, but all three are in Group 2.

One scientific study found that patients taking 400 mg of vitamin B2 (23,000 times the U.S. recommended daily allowance) often found benefit in reducing migraine frequency, severity, and/or duration after three to four months of steady use. No one knows the long term safety of doing that, but vitamin B2 is a water soluble vitamin, so any excess is excreted in the urine. Indeed, the only side effect seems to be that vitamin B2 turns the urine bright yellow.

Generally, the effects of riboflavin are not subtle. It may be more likely to be effective in patients with migraine with aura, although this has yet to be confirmed. Still, riboflavin is inexpensive, some patients find a vitamin more acceptable than prescribed medications, and it may work in up to half the patients who try it for migraine prevention. So most of my patients with more than one migraine every month or two generally want to try it.

The evidence that oral magnesium supplementation can prevent migraine is less certain: two of three scientific studies found benefit. One of the two positive studies was a study in using magnesium supplementation to prevent premenstrual migraine, so menstrual migraine may be a good type to try to prevent with magnesium.

There is good evidence that magnesium given intravenously can stop an ongoing migraine around menstruation in someone with low levels of ionized magnesium. This responsiveness correlates with low serum ionized magnesium as opposed to total serum magnesium.

Oral magnesium takes a long time to get into the brain and stabilize, usually one to three months. If it is chelated, it crosses the blood-brain barrier more easily, and doses of 400–600 mg/day for at least three months are required to see benefit. The big problem with magnesium supplementation is that oral magnesium frequently causes diarrhea and gastrointestinal upset.

Some headache doctors believe that magnesium, like riboflavin, is more likely to work in people with migraine with aura, and as noted above, in women with migraine associated with menstruation.

Feverfew grows wild in many places in the U.S. It is sold over the counter as a dried leaf preparation, usually in a capsule.

A recent review of all the studies on feverfew could not determine if it is effective in migraine prevention. It can cause ulcers in the mouth and loss of the sense of taste, and some people get something similar to withdrawal symptoms of achiness when they stop it.

It rarely causes significant side effects that we know of, but the true potency of the dried-leaf capsules is uncertain. As noted earlier, due to the 1994 Dietary Supplement Health and Education Act, there is no governmental oversight of either safety or potency. I must say I have not been too impressed by the power of feverfew to prevent migraine.

Groups 3, 4, 5, and Beyond

These medications are of two sorts. Those in Group 3 are used widely for migraine prevention and are believed likely to be effective, but no studies have been done to establish their effectiveness. The medications in Group 4 are established by scientific studies to be effective, but the side effects of the medications can be significant. Group 5 medications are those for which evidence suggests they do not prevent migraine. Finally, botulinum toxin and topiramate have been found to be effective subsequent to the governmental literature evidence review.

Ergots—methylergonovine, ergonovine, and DHE

Ergots are discussed in chapter 6. Many of them can be used in migraine prevention, including methylergonovine (Methergine), which is in Group 3b, and ergonovine maleate, which is not rated in any group.

All ergots have one very odd, fortunately rare, and potentially life-threatening side effect. If used on a daily basis for long periods of time, some people will develop scar tissue formation around or in the heart, on the heart valves (similar to what occurred with the diet medication phen/fen), in the lungs, or in the gut. This is called a fibrotic complication and is discussed in chapter 6. Most headache specialists suggest a drug holiday every six months for patients using methylergonovine.

Ergonovine is not available in the U.S., but works about the same as methylergonovine and is closely related. Ergonovine is available in Europe and can be imported for personal use.

Some people who are nauseated with one of these medications may be able to tolerate another, but both can cause the same fibrotic problem. Both can cause the Raynaud's phenomenon and coronary artery narrowing mentioned in chapter 6.

DHE (Group 4) is available in Europe in oral forms, both short-acting and long-acting. The long-acting tablets can be used preventively for migraine as well, but the DHE is not very well absorbed.

Significant concern exists about combining ergots with triptans. If a patient is taking a daily ergot such as methylergonovine to prevent migraines, and gets a breakthrough migraine, it may be dangerous to treat with a triptan. We do not know if the ergot and the triptan working together narrow the coronary arteries to a dangerous degree.

Using an ergot as a preventive medication limits what can be taken safely to get rid of an acute migraine, and poses a risk of life-threatening scar tissue formation if the ergot prevention is used continuously for longer than six months. That is why I prescribe ergot medication less and less to prevent migraine.

Monoamine oxidase inhibitors (MAOIs)

Monoamine oxidase inhibitors (MAOIs) are old-fashioned antidepressants that can be useful in reducing the frequency of migraine. Phenelzine (Nardil) is in Group 3b; tranylcypromine (Parnate) is not even rated in a group, but that is primarily due to a lack of good studies, because headache specialists have known for years that both are effective.

MAOIs work by inhibiting the enzymatic breakdown of monoamines such as adrenaline and serotonin. By increasing adrenaline or serotonin because it is not broken down, patients get increased energy taking MAOIs, sometimes to the point of causing insomnia.

MAOIs can cause weight gain, trouble urinating, and trouble achieving an orgasm. But the biggest problem is that they inhibit the breakdown of the amino acid tyramine, a building block of serotonin and adrenaline. Ingestion of tyramine-containing foods, in the presence of a medication that blocks monoaminime oxidase, can result in hypertension and even cerebral hemorrhage.

Therefore, when taking a MAOI, a restricted diet is required involving the avoidance of foods, beverages, or drugs that contain tyramine or that have adrenaline or serotonin effects. Foods and beverages to avoid include aged, smoked, or fermented foods, pickled foods, sour cream and yogurt, bananas, chicken livers, avocado, soy sauce, broad beans, yeast extracts, dry sausages and prepared meats, chocolate, alcohol beverages, and high caffeine drinks. Among the most important medications to avoid are over-the-counter cold medications such as pseudoephedrine (Sudafed); meperidine (Demerol); SSRI antidepressants such as fluoxetine (Prozac), sertraline (Zoloft), paroxetine (Paxil), citalopram (Celexa), venlafaxine (Effexor); and, unfortunately, most of the triptans (but not naratriptan, frovatriptan, or eletriptan). Given the restricted diet with the risk of serious consequences to a dietary indiscretion or a medicine error, the medication limitations including triptans, and the availability of safer alternatives, I prescribe MAOIs far less often than I did a decade ago.

Antiserotonin medications—cyproheptadine (Periactin), pizotifen

A number of migraine preventive medications appear to block the serotonin-2 or $5\text{-}HT_2$ receptors, the excitatory receptors that may turn on migraine (see chapter 4). The ergots such as methylergonovine and ergonovine may work by blocking $5\text{-}HT_2$, but there are a few other medications that may work by doing so as well.

Cyproheptadine (Periactin) is an old-fashioned antihistamine similar to over-the-counter antihistamines like diphenhydramine (Benadryl) and chlorpheniramine (Chlor-Trimeton). The side effects of cyproheptadine are almost identical to those of the over-the-counter medications, and also to those of the tricyclic antidepressants: drowsiness, dry mouth, constipation, and weight gain.

Inexpensive and safe, cyproheptadine can be a helpful extra medication for co-pharmacy prevention of migraine. It rarely works alone.

Another anti-5HT$_2$ medication, pizotifen (Sandomigran), is listed in Group 4 even though it is not available in the U.S. It is similar to cyproheptadine in every way, but sometimes weight gain will occur with one but not the other, or the drowsiness from one will be less than with the other. Since it is inexpensive, some people arrange to import it for personal use from Canada, Europe, or Latin America.

ACE inhibitors and SSRIs

Angiotensin converting enzyme (ACE) inhibitors and angiotasin receptor blockers (ARBs) reduce blood pressure by inhibiting an enzyme that regulates fluid retention and blood pressure. Rarely, ACE inhibitors cause cough (ARBs do not), but are usually without side effects. ACE inhibitors include captropril (Capoten), lisinopril (Zestril, Prinivil), and enalapril (Vasotec), among others. A few reports suggest that ACE inhibitors may prevent migraine in some people, and recently a small study suggested that the ARB candesartan (Atacand) may also work.

Serotonin specific reuptake inhibitors increase the amount of serotonin available to a patient by suppressing the pump that removes serotonin from the synapse after it has been released. Researchers and patients hoped that serotonin specific reuptake inhibitor antidepressants would be effective in migraine prevention. These include fluoxetine (Prozac), sertraline (Zoloft), paroxetine (Paxil), fluvoxamine (Luvox), citalopram (Celexa), escitalopram (Lexapro), and venlafaxine (Effexor). Another set of related antidepressants, trazodone (Desyrel) and nefazodone (Serzone), are similar.

The AHCPR report concluded that there was not good evidence to support most of them in preventing migraine, although two of them, fluvoxamine and paroxetine, did make it into Group 3a, and fluoxetine is in Group 2. Some atypical related medications that are not usually useful in preventing migraine also made it into Group 3a, including mirtazepine (Remeron), venlafaxine, and trazodone.

The best American scientific study on fluoxetine did not find it effective in reducing the frequency of occasional migraine, although it was effective in reducing daily headache. A recent Italian study once again raised the possibility that it is effective, but it took four months to work. Despite this meager and contradictory data, SSRIs continue to be prescribed widely for migraine prevention.

Fluoxetine provides the best evidence for reducing daily headache that is not rebound. The daily headache that can be helped by fluoxetine includes chronic tension-type headache and transformed or chronic migraine without medication overuse (see chapter 8).

Botulinum toxin and topiramate

Botulinum toxin (Botox, Myobloc), injected into the face, head, and neck, can prevent migraine in more than 50% of patients. Botulinum toxin works by preventing the release of acetylcholine, the neurotransmitter most involved in muscular movement. It may also prevent the release of neurotransmitters that mediate pain, explaining its effectiveness in both migraine prevention and other pain syndromes.

Botulinum toxin must be injected every three months to maintain effectiveness. There are no significant side effects with it.

Topiramate (Topamax) is an anti-epilepsy medication that prevents migraine in at least 50% of patients. Its mechanism of action is quite unclear; as with other effective anti-seizure medications, it probably suppresses central nervous system hyperexcitability. Side effects can include confusion, word-finding difficulty, kidney stones, limb tingling, glaucoma, and weight loss. Three large controlled trials have shown it unequivocally effective, and on the basis of this recent evidence, it belongs in Group I. Official FDA approval of topiramate as a migraine preventive medication is expected in 2003. Because topiramate is effective and can cause weight loss, it is being increasingly used for prevention of migraine.

Mini-prevention of Migraine

It may not always be necessary to take daily medication to prevent migraine. It may be possible to take a drug several days before a time when migraine is predictable, such as a menstrual period. This is considered a mini-prevention treatment, and it works best if there is a known trigger or vulnerable time for migraine.

One widely used example is to take one of the NSAIDs before a menstrual cycle. Conventionally, people will take naproxen sodium two or three times per day beginning two to three days before the expected first day of the menstrual migraine. This sometimes will prevent the migraines or help lessen them, as well as reduce cramps.

Ergots can also be used to prevent migraine, and in the past ergotamine and even DHE have been used the night before the expected first day of menstrual migraine, and then taken for several days. Some people can tolerate other preventive medications for several days before a known trigger.

Medications that can be used briefly in a lucky few include beta blockers, calcium channel blockers, tricyclics, and divalproex. Studies have suggested that sumatriptan, naratriptan, and frovatriptan can also help prevent menstrual migraine.

Headache doctors have been interested in whether triptans might prevent other migraines with known triggers if simpler measures have failed. For a person who always gets a migraine when flying, and for whom an NSAID at the gate before boarding does not work, a triptan or ergot might be worth a try.

8. Other Headaches

Episodic Tension-type Headache

Episodic tension-type headache is the ordinary headache that most of us get from time to time. It is generally mild, dull, on both sides of the head, and not throbbing. It is often not even worth taking medication for, and usually short-lived, without nausea or other features. The International Headache Society has developed criteria for diagnosing episodic tension-type headaches:

1. The patient should have had at least ten of these headaches.
2. The headaches last from 30 minutes to seven days.
3. The headaches must have at least two of the following four:
   a. Non-throbbing quality
   b. Mild or moderate intensity, either not affecting activity, or inhibiting without prohibiting activity
   c. Two-sided location
   d. No aggravation by routine physical activity such as bending over or climbing stairs
4. Both of the following:
   a. No nausea or vomiting
   b. Absence of dislike of noise or light
5. Less than 15 days of headache per month and less than 180 days per year.
6. Secondary causes are excluded.

The reason that the woman in chapter 1 with moderate menstrual headache does not fit the diagnosis of episodic tension-type headache is the presence of worsening pain when she bent over, and dislike of both noise and light. And yet both patients and doctors alike might call that headache a tension or stress headache.

Using the IHS criteria can be helpful in not missing a migraine diagnosis. However, for the most part, when a headache is annoying enough to complain about, it is migraine and not tension-type headache.

Episodic tension-type headache is common, with low disability. But, because so many people have it, the cost to society is not inconsiderable.

Chronic Daily Headache

Daily headache is divided for diagnostic purposes into short and long—that is, daily headaches lasting less than and more than four hours a day.

Daily or frequent headache is not uncommon. Recent studies in several countries around the world have found that 4–5% of people have daily or near daily headache. Most of these people have long daily headaches. Headaches lasting less than four hours a day but occurring every day are much more rare.

Short-lasting Daily Headaches

Short-lasting headaches are ice-pick pains, SUNCT (Short-lasting Unilateral Neuralgiform headaches with Conjunctival injection and Tearing), EPH/CPH (Episodic and Chronic Paroxysmal Hemicrania), and cluster. All of these headaches are relatively rare, so I recommend that all people with them get a careful neurologic exam and at least one imaging study of the head—either a CAT scan or an MRI scan—because other secondary disorders (see chapter 1) can masquerade as these relatively rare types of headaches.

Idiopathic stabbing headache (ice-pick pain, jabs and jolts syndrome)
The shortest of the short headaches are the stabbing headaches. These are described by people as sharp, needlelike jabs that feel like an ice pick. They can occur alone or in volleys of jabs.

They occur in up to 40% of people with migraine, often in the usual location of the migraine. A single ice-pick pain will occur now and then, usually occurring so fast that it cannot be treated.

However, if there is a series of jabs and jolts, treatment is recommended. Sometimes, a series of stabs will lead up to a migraine, and the entire episode can be stopped.

It turns out that there is an effective medication treatment, but only one. It is the NSAID indomethacin (Indocin). Indomethacin turns off idiopathic stabbing headaches like a key in a lock. Why ice-pick pain and other short-lasting daily headaches respond only to indomethacin is one of the great mysteries of headache.

Indomethacin actually works for many forms of short headache. Not all short headaches respond to indomethacin, but those that do respond absolutely. They are referred to as "indomethacin-responsive headaches."

I usually start my patients on the smallest dose of indomethacin available, 25 mg, three times a day with meals. Each form of indomethacin-responsive headache can take up to a week to respond to the proper dose of indomethacin, so I have my patients take that dose for one full week to see if it works before moving up the dose. If there is a partial response at lower doses of indomethacin, it is worth increasing the dose.

Indomethacin can have side effects similar to other NSAIDs. In particular, gastrointestinal upset such as heartburn or nausea can be a problem. These can sometimes be minimized by using a low dose and taking the drug with food, but patients with a history of gastroesophageal reflux disease or ulcers rarely tolerate it. Occasionally, people who cannot take oral indomethacin can take a suppository form or a liquid, but this is usually not necessary.

Use of indomethacin over a long time can cause kidney problems, a problem shared by all anti-inflammatories. As noted in chapter 7, NSAIDs also can cause bleeding problems and ulcers. Very rarely, indomethacin can cause eye problems, so I also recommend yearly eye checks by an ophthalmologist for those taking regular indomethacin.

SUNCT

The next form of short-lasting headaches—fortunately the most rare, because they have not been found to respond reliably to any treatment—are called short-lasting unilateral neuralgiform headaches with conjunctival injection and tearing or SUNCT headaches.

These headaches last only a few seconds, but usually longer than ice-pick pains. They are also sharp in quality, occur on only one side behind the eye, and are accompanied by the eye immediately turning red and tearing.

The technical term for short headaches with eye and nose symptoms is trigeminal-autonomic cephalalgias, or TACs. As quickly as SUNCT headaches arrive, they disappear, but they occur over and over again every day. They hurt terribly but no completely effective treatment is known.

Episodic and chronic paroxysmal hemicranias (EPH/CPH)

The next type of daily headaches that last less than four hours per day and respond to indomethacin are the paroxysmal hemicranias. These headaches are usually short, lasting about 30 minutes. They are almost always on the same side of the head, and occur many times per day. These short headaches happen more than five times per day more than half the time.

The pain of the paroxysmal hemicranias is usually sharp and not throbbing. The headaches are associated with similar symptoms to SUNCT. That is, the eye can turn red and tear, as with other TACs. Other symptoms that can occur in the paroxysmal hemicranias at the time of the headaches are stuffy nose, runny nose, forehead and facial sweating, small pupil, droopy eyelid, or eyelid swelling. One or all of these symptoms can be present at the time of the attack.

As stated above, the headache attacks occur often every day. Sometimes they go away for months or years at a time, only to return. That condition is called episodic paroxysmal hemicrania or EPH.

Other people get the attacks every day, and they never go away. These people have chronic paroxysmal hemicrania, or CPH.

The good news is that both forms respond absolutely to indomethacin, used as described above. As always with indomethacin, when it works it works completely. No one really understands the causes of EPH/CPH, no one understands why some people go long periods without the headaches and other people get them every day with stopping, and no one understands why indomethacin works so, completely—but it is remarkable when it kicks in.

I remember the first person I saw with CPH as a medical student at Cornell University Medical College in New York City. The man had 20 headaches per day and had not worked in years, due to the severity and frequency of his headaches. After being given daily indomethacin, he stopped having his headaches, went back to work, and told us that his life had been given back to him.

Trigeminal neuralgia (tic douloreux)

Trigeminal neuralgia or tic douloreux is a disorder of fierce, brief, lightning-like pains, generally across the face. These are often triggered by a specific movement or event, such as brushing the teeth, eating, or wind on the face.

The likely cause of trigeminal neuralgia is a series of abnormal electrical discharges along the trigeminal nerve, a cranial nerve exiting from the brainstem and serving sensation on the face. The cause of the discharges can be an aberrant blood vessel looping over the nerve and putting pressure on the nerve, or an injury to the nerve, causing irritability. The discharges, which are analogous to an epileptic seizure of this nerve, can usually be suppressed with anti-seizure medications such as carbamazepine (Tegretol), oxcarbazepine (Trileptal), or gabapentin (Neurontin). Occasionally, surgery is necessary to stop the pains.

Sometimes it is hard to tell trigeminal neuralgia from ice-pick pain, but the former is usually much more severe and does not respond to indomethacin. As with all the short headaches, I recommend an imaging study before the diagnosis is made.

Cluster

Cluster headaches are also a rare form of short-lasting daily headaches, or TACs, and occur in less than one percent of people.

This form of headache occurs more frequently in men, about four times as often as in women.

A cluster headache is a severe pain centered on one side, usually behind the eye or temple. The pain is sharp or boring, like a hot poker piercing the eye, and is one of the most terrible forms of headache pain.

The headache attacks are brief, lasting 15 minutes to three hours, but usually about an hour. They are longer than other TACs. Cluster attacks occur about one to three times per day, although sometimes as often as eight in a day.

Unlike in migraine where people want to lie still, during an attack a cluster patient may be agitated and constantly pace.

Cluster headache attacks can occur at the same time every day or each night. They are sometimes called "alarm clock headaches."

Cluster headache patients experience one or more of the same symptoms at the time of the headache on the same side of the head listed above for the other TACs (SUNCT and EPH/CPH): red eye, tearing, nasal stuffiness, runny nose, droopy eyelid, small pupil, eyelid swelling, and/or forehead and facial sweating.

Cluster headache attacks generally occur daily or near daily for two to three months and then, like EPH, they go away for months or years. When a person is having daily cluster headache attacks, the time period of the daily headaches is called a cluster period. A person who has cluster attacks, then periods without attacks, then periods with attacks again is said to have episodic cluster headaches, similar to EPH (but usually not responsive to indomethacin).

Some unfortunate people have cluster attacks every day but do not have periods without cluster attacks; they are felt to have chronic cluster headache, similar to CPH. One form of cluster can transform into the other, and, for the lucky few, the disease itself can burn itself out and go away forever.

For reasons that are unclear, not only is cluster more common in men, it is more common in smokers. During a cluster period, the cluster attacks can be triggered by lowered oxygen from a cigarette, but also by alcohol intake, strong fumes, excessive exercise, and napping or extra sleep.

The exact causes of cluster headache have not yet been determined. Cluster was originally considered a variant of migraine, but a dramatic difference lies in the central brain generators for migraine versus cluster. In migraine, the central generator was photographed on PET scans turning on in the upper brainstem.

In cluster, the central generator is located in the hypothalamus. Since the hypothalamus is the area of the brain that regulates cycles such as day/night, this explains the circadian rhythm of cluster.

Cluster headaches, whether episodic or chronic, require both daily preventive treatment and acute or abortive treatment.

Acute treatment of cluster

Oxygen works very well. This is unique in headache: an adequate abortive treatment is breathing oxygen at a rate of 7 to 8 liters/minute through a re-breathing mask from an oxygen tank during an attack while sitting, bending forward, and looking at the floor. The oxygen usually stops the attacks in 20 minutes or less. It works even better if the patient is on good preventive medication.

The drawback of treatment with oxygen is that it is not easily portable. Many patients use oxygen for attacks at home, and other medications for attacks occurring at work or away from home. The mechanism of action of oxygen is a mystery.

Triptans also work in aborting a cluster attack. Specifically, sumatriptan 6 mg injection is extremely effective in stopping cluster within 30 minutes, and is approved by the FDA for this purpose. Sumatriptan injection comes in the handy statdose system or autoinjector for carrying out of the house. However, it is more expensive and has more side effects than oxygen (see chapter 6). Recently, sumatriptan nasal spray was found to abort cluster headaches.

Zolmitriptan in pill form has been shown to be effective in stopping cluster attacks. The attack must be at least 45 minutes long; the dose is 5 mg or 10 mg of zolmitriptan, higher than the 2.5 mg dose with which we start migraine patients.

Ergots also abort cluster attacks. DHE can be given by self-injection, but there is no autoinjector device. Ergotamine can work in suppository form, but most people do not want to use it.

Preventive treatment of cluster

Verapamil, ergotamine, lithium, and/or divalproex are commonly used for preventive treatment of cluster headache. I often use multiple medications at once, instead of a single preventive drug. The co-pharmacy allows me to use lower doses, and successfully treat a higher percentage of cluster patients.

I start with **verapamil**. This calcium channel blocker is described in chapter 6. In migraine patients we use long-acting verapamil once or twice per day, but in cluster patients short-acting verapamil at 80 mg three times per day may work better. The side effects of constipation and foot swelling are sometimes a problem, and the drug needs to be used carefully, if at all, in patients with heart disease.

Often another medication is needed on a daily basis to stop the cluster attacks. **Lithium carbonate** can be used. I recommend 300 mg three times a day. Lithium can affect the kidneys and the thyroid and requires blood checks. It can cause thirst, a bad taste in the mouth, tremor, and weight gain. As with oxygen, lithium is effective in cluster but not in most other headache types.

Other medications that can be added to verapamil or to verapamil plus lithium, are the anti-epilepsy drugs **divalproex**, **topiramate**, or **gabapentin**, which are covered in chapter 7.

Ergotamine, taken nightly, is helpful in preventing cluster, and unlike in migraine, it does not cause rebound headache. Side effects include nausea and Raynaud's, and people on ergotamine daily cannot take triptans.

Steroids such as prednisone are used to prevent cluster, but can only be used for a couple of weeks, and other preventive medications need to be on board when the prednisone is stopped.

Prednisone causes the full gamut of steroid effects: stomach upset and ulcers, sleep disturbance and insomnia, acne and weight gain, altered mood, and alterations of potassium and sodium levels in the blood. Since steroids can alter immune response, only short courses of treatment are suggested.

Another possible treatment for prevention of cluster is to use **capsaicin**, a derivative of the active ingredient of hot peppers, administered daily by paste or liquid in the nose on the side of the cluster attack. Because most people do not want to do this, a synthetic form similar to capsaicin (**civamide**) is being studied. It is a sign of the severity of the pain of cluster that patients are willing to undertake this type of treatment.

Long-lasting Daily Headaches

The next types of daily headaches last longer than four hours a day and are divided into hemicrania continua, new daily persistent headache, chronic tension-type headache, and the most important, transformed or chronic migraine.

Hemicrania continua

Hemicrania continua is a rare but treatable form of long-lasting daily headache. The headache in this disorder is always on one side of the head, is continuous, and is present most if not all of the time.

Hemicrania continua is usually a mild to moderate daily headache, but superimposed on daily moderate, one-sided headaches can be episodes of more severe headache occurring on the same side as the daily headache and having the characteristics of migraine. The more severe exacerbations can last from 45 minutes to days.

People with hemicrania continua can have other symptoms associated with their headaches. They can have ice-pick pains on the same side. Dr. Larry Newman and Dr. Richard Lipton of Albert Einstein School of Medicine described people with hemicrania continua as having a gritty sensation or the sensation of a foreign body in the eye on the side of the headache. Some people will have the same symptoms on the same side as occur in cluster headaches, EPH/CPH, or other TACs.

The diagnosis of hemicrania continua is made certain by a complete response to indomethacin. This makes this condition similar to ice-pick pains and EPH/CPH. Once again, the indomethacin is a key in the lock, and fully eliminates the headache.

What causes this headache is unknown. Since some patients seem to develop it after having experienced migraine, perhaps there is a relationship between the two headache types; but of course migraine is not 100% treatable with indomethacin, so the relationship is still unclear. The disorder is rare enough that I always make sure a patient has a CAT or MRI scan as part of the work-up.

New daily persistent headache

Some people with daily headache can state exactly when their headaches began, sometimes to the date and time. If they have never had headaches before and there is no secondary cause for their headaches, such as trauma or disease, they are said to have "new daily persistent headache."

Some of these patients have had a viral infection that has resulted in the problem; these headaches were originally called "post-viremic headaches." In either case, the result is the same: headaches for more than four hours a day for more than one month in a row without an obvious secondary cause.

Treatment can be very difficult. As with most forms of primary long-lasting daily headaches, studies on treatment are few and most are not very impressive. Most medications for daily headache do not work more than 40% of the time in the well-done studies, and regular aerobic exercise and other non-drug therapies seem to work at about that level as well. For this reason, I always encourage my patients with daily headache to start with regular aerobic exercise.

One study on fluoxetine (Prozac) published in 1994 suggested that it prevented these daily headaches. In that study, depressed patients were not included, so the effect of the fluoxetine was not on depression. I often try fluoxetine for my patients once I am certain that there are no other causes for daily headaches to be found, and if exercise has not worked.

The dose in the study was 40 mg per day, and the drug usually took three months to work, so it is a long haul. Side effects of fluoxetine can include excessive activation or agitation up to and including insomnia, upset stomach with nausea and diarrhea, weight loss, and sexual problems, including decreased libido, impotence, and trouble achieving orgasm.

Other SSRIs have also been described as effective in long, chronic daily headache, specifically paroxetine.

Medications working at the 40% level also include amitriptyline and tricyclic antidepressants, divalproex, and gabapentin (see chapter 7). Recently, botulinum toxin has been described as working for an even higher percentage of daily-headache patients.

Chronic tension-type headache

Some people get tension-type headaches every day. Chronic tension-type headache is a continuous low-grade, two-sided headache that often develops in people who previously had the episodic tension-type headache discussed at the beginning of this chapter. Treatment is identical to that described above for new daily persistent headache, and involves trying regular aerobic exercise and biofeedback training, sometimes with fluoxetine and other medications.

The IHS has developed the following diagnostic criteria for chronic tension-type headache:

1. Headache at least 15 days a month for at least six months
2. At least two of the following:
   a. Non-throbbing pain
   b. Mild or moderate severity which either does not affect or mildly inhibits, but does not prohibit, activity
   c. Two-sided location
   d. Headache pain not worsened by routine physical activity such as climbing stairs or bending over
3. Both of the following:
   e. No vomiting
   f. None of the following:
      i. Nausea (or mild nausea only)
      ii. Dislike of light
      iii. Dislike of noise
4. Normal exam findings or imaging study such as CAT or MRI scan

Transformed and Chronic migraine

A current theory is that, as some people with episodic tension-type headache can transform gradually into chronic tension-type headache, so too can people with episodic migraine transform into sufferers of chronic daily migraine.

Proposed criteria for this transformed migraine include some of the following:

1. Headache occurring at least 15 days per month for at least one month, lasting at least four hours per day if untreated
2. A previous history of episodic migraine headaches
3. A period of transformation during which, for some people, the frequency of all headache increases, while the frequency of severe or migrainous headache may decrease
4. Migraines that occur daily or near daily instead of lasting 4–72 hours

Dr. Richard Lipton of New York and Dr. Steven Silberstein of Jefferson Medical School of Philadelphia further note that all the common daily long-lasting headaches—chronic tension-type headache, new daily persistent headache, and chronic migraine—can come in two forms: those occurring in people taking no medication, and those associated with taking too much medication. Chronic tension-type headaches and transformed migraines without medication overuse evolve slowly but spontaneously out of the intermittent or episodic forms; for the forms associated with medication overuse to change into a daily or near daily form of headache, a person must dose with medications frequently. This transformation by relief medications or transformed migraine with medication overuse is also called rebound headache. It is very common in people with migraine and is the most common cause of frequent headache. Table 8.1 lists some of the medications that can cause rebound headache, also called medication overuse headache (MOH).

There are several important points about rebound headache, besides how often it occurs. When a patient is in rebound, no other medication works for headache except the drug from which withdrawal is occurring on a daily basis. The rebound medications do not keep a patient headache free, either.

Table 8.1 Some medications that can cause rebound Over the counter medications (6–10/week)
Analgesics aspirin, acetaminophen (Tylenol), ibuprofen (Advil, Motrin), naproxen sodium (Aleve), ketoprofen (Orudis)
Mixed analgesics Bufferin, Excedrin, Anacin, Vanquish, BC powder, Goody's powder
Nasal decongestants pseudoephedrine (Sudafed), oxymetazoline (Afrin), phenylpropanolamine
Antihistamines diphenhydramine (Benadryl), chlorpheniramine, dimenhydrinate, meclizine
Mixed cold and allergy medications Chlor-Trimeton, Tristan, Dimetapp, Drixoral, Comtrex, Coricidin D, Contac, Actifed, Sine-aid, Sinutab
Sleeping medications diphenhydramine (Sominex, Unisom, Nytol)
Caffeine
Prescription medications (2–3 days/week)
Analgesics Tramadol, propoxyphene, codeine, hydrocodone, oxydodone, hydromorphone, oxymorphone, morphine, methadone, fentanyl, butorphanol
NSAIDs Ibuprofen, naproxen, fenoprofen, flurbiprofen, ketoprofen, mefanamic acid, meclofenamate, ketorolac
Tranquilizers butalbital, diazepam, alprazolam, clonazepam, triazolam, lorazepam, zolpidem
Ergots ergotamine, DHE
Triptans all

Medications prescribed to prevent headache usually do not work when a patient is taking frequent relief medications and having daily or near daily headaches. Even the powerful migraine-specific medications such as triptans either will not work or will relieve the headaches only briefly during rebound. People with this problem often come into my office with a long list of medications that they have tried unsuccessfully.

Importantly, medications that fail to work on someone taking relief medications frequently will work, once the relief medications have been discontinued. Stopping excessive use of relief medications is the important first step in the road back from daily headache to migraine in discrete episodes. This is truly a detoxification.

This detoxification can take up to seven months, but people usually feel better and have less headache within several weeks of stopping all of their immediate-relief medications. However, I do not recommend stopping these medications cold turkey without help; this will almost assuredly result in a rip-roaring withdrawal headache, and sometimes a full-blown migraine.

Of equal importance, there has never been a reported case of a person getting better from rebound headache without stopping the medications that cause the headaches.

There are multiple theories on the causes of transformed migraine with medication overuse. One is that rebound is habituation and withdrawal: a patient habituated to a medication will experience withdrawal symptoms such as headache in a regular daily pattern.

A second theory suggests that overuse of medications leads to brain toxicity, possibly mediated by free-radical formation (release of charged particles that damage the neuronal tissue), resulting in chronic pain. A third theory is that overuse of medication causes an increase in 5-HT_2 excitatory serotonin receptors, with chronic migraine as a result.

People with rebound headache often receive poor treatment by their caregivers and friends and loved ones. Because this is a common problem, it is worth examining.

First, MOH is a common problem. Several studies have shown that the frequency of headache greater than 15 days a month is about 4–5% in the general population. Of these people, about half have chronic tension-type headache, and half have chronic migraine, usually rebound.

When doctors, nurse practitioners, physician assistants, and other caregivers are confronted with a person with daily headache, they often reach to try to find other causes for the daily headache, such as a "bad neck" or "muscle contraction" or temporomandibular joint (TMJ) dysfunction. This list can go on and on. Instead, there should be an attempt to establish a previous history of episodic headache and over-use of medications.

Remember that it only takes a couple of aspirin, Excedrin, or acetaminophen (Tylenol) a day to give a headache person rebound daily headache.

Friends and loved ones, too, often blame the person with the daily headaches. Acquaintances will frequently have their own theories as to the "cause" for the daily headaches, such as something in the diet or in the environment, or they will have a "magic cure," such as a new herb, supplement, operation, or gadget.

If medication overuse is suggested, caregivers, patients, and their friends and loved ones will sometimes misinterpret this to mean addiction. But rebound is not addiction. Addiction is a social problem and behavior in which people seek medication.

Most people with rebound are inadvertently habituated, not addicted. All they need is directions in how to detoxify and go back over the bridge to migraine in discrete episodes.

Treatment of rebound

There are several ways to successfully detoxify and get out of the loop. Some people can do it outside the hospital; others require a hospitalization.

There are two ways to get out of rebound as an outpatient, one slow and one fast.

In the slow approach, I take the following steps with my patients:

1. Together we select one or more preventive medications for migraine and begin them slowly, increasing them every four to seven days until the patient is on an adequate dose of the preventive medication.
2. We start a slow taper of the immediate-relief rebound medications. For example, if the patient is taking two Fiorinal and two Excedrin a day, I write out the taper: Week one, take one Fiorinal and two Excedrin per day; Week two, take one Fiorinal and one Excedrin per day, and so forth, down by a tablet per day per week.

3. I provide some relief medications, generally triptans (unless the patient is rebounding from triptans), and limit their use to no more than two days per week and then only to treat severe headache. After a few weeks, I tell my patients not to treat any mild or moderate headache.

4. Once the patient is off the rebound medications, it usually takes one to three months for the episodic migraine pattern to reappear. I see them monthly to adjust medication, answer questions and give encouragement.

5. After they have settled into a pattern of migraine in discrete episodes without daily headache for three to six months on daily preventive medication, I usually try tapering off the daily medication. Patients often can come off of daily preventive medications and treat only the occasional migraine with triptans on an irregular basis.

To do outpatient detoxification the quick way, I start my patient on preventive medication and abruptly stop the rebound medications. If they are not in rebound from a triptan, I start them on sumatriptan 25–50 mg three times a day for ten days as a bridge, or until they are headache free for 24 hours.

When the ten days are up, or when they get 24 hours of headache freedom, it is important to stop the repetitive use of sumatriptan to avoid developing dependence and rebound from it.

The sumatriptan helps treat the withdrawal headaches and serves as a bridge through the detoxification. If the headaches get very bad, the patient can take extra sumatriptan. Once through the withdrawal period, the patient can continue to use sumatriptan to treat occasional migraines. Other medications such as steroids, NSAIDs, and nasal DHE can also be used as a bridge through the withdrawal.

This approach can be done only if stopping cold turkey off the rebound medication is not going to cause a serious problem. If the patient is taking a lot of Fiorinal, which contains a barbiturate, or an anxiety-reducing tranquilizer or sleeper such as Ambien (zolpidem), Xanax (alprazolam), Ativan (lorazepam), Valium (diazepam), Klonopin (clonazepam), or similar medication, an abrupt discontinuation can be dangerous, causing withdrawal seizures or worse. For this reason, rebound detoxification requires medical supervision.

If outpatient detoxification has been tried unsuccessfully, a patient is on a lot of medications, has other medical problems, or is on medications that are dangerous to withdraw from, an inpatient approach to detoxification should be followed. This involves the following steps:

1. On day 1 in the hospital, preventive medications for migraine are started.
2. The rebound medications are either abruptly stopped or tapered safely and quickly, sometimes using other medications at the same time.
3. Intravenous antinauseant medication and DHE are both administered, sometimes with intravenous ketorolac, valproate, or steroids, on a regular schedule until the patient is headache free. These intravenous medications treat the withdrawal headaches and withdrawal symptoms and also serve as a bridge to detoxification.
4. Once headache free, the patient is discharged from the hospital, on daily preventive medications and detoxified from rebound medications. The patient is given a prescription for a migraine specific medication (usually a triptan or DHE in injectable or nasal form, such as Migranal) to use for discrete episodes of migraine, not more than two days per week.

This approach is known as the DHE protocol; over 90% of these patients with rebound are headache free within three days. The long-term outlook is also good, with at least two-thirds of patients maintaining their good outcome, meaning an occasional migraine but not daily headache.

Once again, if a patient is doing well after three to six months of daily preventive medication, with occasional migraine, I try to taper the daily preventive medication to see if they can use migraine-specific medication, such as a triptan or DHE, only as needed.

The outlook for most rebound sufferers is excellent. Detoxification usually restores an intermittent headache pattern. Although the patient is likely to still have an occasional migraine, the migraines are treatable. Once detoxified, daily headache usually disappears, and an occasional migraine is a much more acceptable situation than daily headache, easier to treat and less disabling.

Headaches Associated with Sex, Exercise, and Cough

Another rare headache type is significant headache associated with sexual activity. The usual situation is to have an explosive headache, like a migraine, at or near orgasm.

Occasionally, the new onset of this type of headache is a sign of an aneurysm in the brain giving a warning bleed before a full-blown hemorrhage. Therefore a work-up may include a CAT scan, a magnetic resonance angiogram (MRA), or even a spinal tap. An invasive study of brain arteries in the hospital (4-vessel angiogram) may be necessary.

If there is no aneurysm, or if sexual headaches have occurred for many years, this is the benign type of this disorder. Sometimes this headache can be prevented with indomethacin taken an hour before sexual activity, making this type of headache yet another indomethacin-responsive headache.

Another headache that sometimes raises the question of aneurysm is migraine precipitated by exercise or weight lifting. The benign type is also called "effort migraine." It, too, can sometimes be prevented by taking indomethacin an hour before exercise.

Cough headache is a short headache that occurs with cough, bowel movement, or, occasionally, weight lifting. Unlike effort migraine, it is extremely brief, a short "pow," and then a quick resolution. This headache peaks virtually instantly, rarely lasting longer than 30 seconds.

Cough headache can sometimes be a symptom of an abnormality in the brain, called a Chiari malformation, where a part of the cerebellum at the back of the brain hangs too low, herniating from the brain into the spinal cord. A Chiari malformation can sometimes require surgical correction, so it is important to make the diagnosis. Anyone with onset of cough headache requires an MRI of the junction of the brainstem and the neck.

The benign form of cough headache can be treated preventively with daily indomethacin in the usual manner. Sometimes, benign cough headache can be cured with a spinal tap in which a large amount of spinal fluid is removed. This works in about half of the patients treated, not as high a success rate as with oral indomethacin, but without the need for daily medication. Cough headache often resolves spontaneously in several years.

The causes of sex and exercise headaches are obscure. Cough headache may be related to increased cerebral spinal fluid volume, explaining its increase with increased intrathoracic pressure from cough or straining at stool (valsalva) and its improvement with fluid reduction via spinal tap.

9. New Areas of Research

Genetics

One area of hot research is the search for a gene or genes for migraine. In chapter 4 I discussed the genes so far found that determine familial hemiplegic migraine (FHM). Those genes code for calcium channels or sodium channels. The question is whether other migraines could be caused by abnormal gates or channels that have problems in regulating how chemicals or molecules get into or out of the nerve cells.

One area of research has demonstrated that there are, in fact, abnormal calcium channel manifestations in other forms of migraine. Clinical signs include subtly abnormal cerebellar incoordination (the cerebellum has a dense distribution of calcium channels), and abnormal motor function (the neuromuscular junction is dependent on calcium channels).

The likelihood of finding signs of calcium channel abnormality increases with the severity of aura: some patients with conventional migraine with aura showed these abnormalities, more with prolonged aura, and even more with hemiplegic aura. Research is ongoing to determine the extent of calcium channel dysfunction in the commoner forms of migraine, and how to find it simply for picking treatment.

Some pharmaceutical companies are creating gene banks to explore migraine patients' genes. So far, though, no other abnormal channels have been found outside of those people with FHM, although recently a sodium channel abnormality gene has been described in FHM.

Another area of genetic research is examination of the genes that code neurotransmitter structure, storage, receptors, and metabolism. The obvious interest is in serotonin, because it is associated with migraine, depression, irritable bowel disease, sleep, and many other co-morbid illnesses. However, other neurotransmitters may also be involved in migraine genetics.

For example, dopamine is a neurotransmitter associated with nausea, and some anti-dopamine drugs, the antinauseants, can turn off migraine in some people. Recent studies have found a group of migraine patients who have a genetic tendency to be too sensitive to dopamine, or to make too much dopamine. And these people have an excessive amount of nausea during their migraines.

The abnormal genes code for the dopamine 2 (or D2) receptor, suggesting a mechanism for this clinical presentation. Study of response to D2 antagonists (such as the new antipsychotic medications risperdone, olanzepine, and quitiapine) and the relationship to D2 genes is the logical next step.

Another potential genetic abnormality involves a complex set of genes that appear to be associated with autoimmune diseases such as rheumatoid arthritis, systemic lupus erythematosis, and Sjogren's syndrome. Clinical studies suggest that migraine occurs more commonly in these diseases.

Here, too, as with the D2 abnormality, subsets of migraine patients may be treatable based on genetic makeup. Studies are in process (but not yet enrolling patients) that match the migraine type, the presence or absence of certain genes, and response to medications for those genetically caused forms of migraine.

For example, the controlled study on riboflavin suggests that there is a group of patients with energy metabolism problems at the level of the cellular organelle, the mitochondrion (see chapter 4). A patient with another group of genes might inherit low ionized magnesium levels and menstrual migraine. The low magnesium would destabilize the nerve membranes, leading to nerves firing too easily.

Another set of genes could code for too much dopamine or sensitivity to dopamine resulting in excessive nausea with migraines; these patients should respond to anti-dopamine drugs. Yet another group of genes could code for abnormal calcium channels, and respond to specific calcium channel blockers. Or there may be a serotonin group of abnormal genes, resulting in the full gamut of abnormal serotonin diseases—migraine, depression, anxiety, insomnia, and irritable bowel disease. A patient might have some or many of these gene sets, or have a mixture. In that scenario, migraine would be like heart disease, where a patient has a set of risk factors that could be tallied up and treated individually or collectively, as is done with risk factors for heart disease.

This offers a potentially exciting future. At least three pharmaceutical companies are trying to match their gene bank data with their medication options. I can see a time when the doctor draws a blood sample for migraine genetic analysis, and the lab tests tell what kind of migraine a patient has and what medications will result in the best response.

Nitric Oxide

Nitric oxide serves as a cellular messenger, causing vasodilation and neuronal excitation (see chapter 4). Neuroscientists believe that abnormally high amounts of nitric oxide can trigger aura or migraine itself. Many of the medications that we use to prevent migraine, such as certain calcium channel blockers, methylergonovine, and cyproheptadine, interfere with the creation or function of nitric oxide—which fits this hypothesis.

A group in Denmark used a medication that inhibited nitric oxide synthesis (L-methylarginine HCl or 546C88) and found in a small study that they could abort acute migraines with this drug. Nitric oxide is synthesized in many tissues, and the genes that regulate it are inducible, meaning they can be switched on or off. Clinical effectiveness most likely will come from inhibiting inducible and neuronal nitric oxide synthase (NOS); further controlled pharmacologic studies of inhibitors of synthesis and function of these two forms of NOS are under way.

Aura and Spreading Depression

Spreading depression and aura have now been linked in studies using functional MRI techniques characterizing the onset, speed, progression, pattern, and duration of and recovery from aura.

Researchers at Harvard Medical School, including Professor Michael Moskowitz and Dr. Michael Cutrer (now at the Mayo Clinic), assumed that blood flow is a useful surrogate for neuronal activation, and studied a patient in whom aura could be induced by exercise. He played basketball at the hospital gym and then raced into the MRI scanner, where his entire aura could be imaged. As occurred in animal models of spreading depression, there was a wave of neuronal excitation with increased blood flow, followed in its wake by a wave of decreased neuronal function spreading forward in the brain at a rate of 3 mm/minute.

The same research group recently were able to connect the spreading depression physiology in animals to the activation of the brain and the vasodilation and inflammation in the meninges. Thus, with the understanding of the physiology of the genesis of the aura so tantalizingly close, blocking the spreading depression may be a key to stopping migraine in patients with aura.

Potential New Treatments for Migraine

Triptans

Donitriptan, a triptan developed in France, is in human studies for efficacy and safety in Europe.

Anti-seizure Medications

Several anti-seizure medications, in addition to divalproex, gabapentin, and topiramate, have shown some promise in preventing migraine. They include levatiracetam (Keppra), zonesamide (Zonegran), and tiagabine (Gabatril).

Controlled studies are under way on levatiracetam, and being contemplated for zonesamide. All three medications are quite safe; drowsiness tends to be the most difficult side effect.

CGRP Antagonists

Calcitonin gene related peptide (CGRP) is the most potent vasodilator in the central nervous system. It is released in migraine neuroinflammatory changes in the meninges. The first controlled study on a specific CGRP antagonist, BIB4096BS, has not been published but has been reported to be effective in migraine.

CGRP antagonism matches clinical efficacy, and several pharmaceutical companies are proceeding with further controlled studies on these medications.

Adenosine A1 Receptors

5-HT_{1B}, 5-HT_{1D}, and adenosine A1 receptors are all receptors in trigeminal neurons in the brainstem. Drugs that activate the A1 receptors (such as GR79236, a GlaxoSmithKline medication) inhibit CGRP release from the neurons that mediate migraine inflammation in the meningeal vasculatrure. Interestingly, these medications also work in the brainstem itself, which could interfere with pain transmission. New A1 antagonists are being planned for controlled studies in the U.S. The major side effect concern with this group of medications is cardiac.

Botulinum Toxin

A series of controlled studies are under way on the effectiveness of botulinum toxin in the prevention of episodic migraine and chronic daily headaches. Areas that remain to be clarified include which sites should be injected, what dose should be used, whether painful areas on the head and neck should be injected, and which patients are candidates for this treatment. Both forms of botulinum toxin, types A and B, are currently being studied.

Anti-Alzheimer Medications

An Italian group has reported that the acetylcholinesterase inhibitor donepezil (Aricept), which is used to treat Alzheimer disease, is effective in preventing migraine. This raises the question whether acetylcholine plays a role in migraine. Since it is inhibited by botulinum toxin, this becomes difficult to understand. They plan further studies.

Appendix: Sources for Information and Support

Resources for People with Migraine

World Headache Alliance
208 Lexington Rd.
Oakville, ON
Canada L6H 6L6
www.w-h-a.org

The World Headache Alliance (WHA) sponsors worldwide initiatives for people with headaches, including educational symposia and outreach programs for many countries. You may want to access this website first; it is a clearinghouse for headache sites and resources, and tries to keep up-to-date information on all phone numbers and addresses.

The American Council for Headache Education
875 Kings Highway, Suite 200
Woodbury, NJ 08096
1-800-255-ACHE
www.achenet.org

One of the major American headache organizations for patients, the American Council (ACHE) is sponsored by the American Headache Society (formerly the American Association for the Study of Headache). ACHE sponsors all sorts of educational opportunities for people with headache—a quarterly ACHE newsletter, a website, and patient support groups. ACHE is in alliance with the WHA and coordinates activities with them.

National Headache Foundation
820 N. Orleans, Suite 217

Chicago, IL 60610-3132
1-800-843-2256
www.headaches.org

The National Headache Foundation (NHF) also has major educational initiatives and programs. The NHF has its own website, newsletter for patients (*NHF Head Lines*) and a network of support groups.

The Migraine Foundation
120 Carlton St., Suite 210
Toronto, ON
Canada M5A 4K2

British Migraine Association
1778A High Rd.
Byfleet, West Byfleet
Surrey, UK
KT14 7ED

The Migraine Trust
45 Great Ormond St.
London, UK
WC1N 3HZ

Websites of Professional Organizations

American Headache Society (formerly American Association for the Study of Headache)
www.AHS.org

National Headache Foundation
www.headaches.org

International Headache Society
www.i-h-s.org

If you want to check on new physician information, these are excellent sites with good links. These organizations also put out journals for specialists: *Headache* (AHS), *Headache and Pain* (NHF), and *Cephalalgia* (IHS). If you want to read the major physician journals on headache, these three are the best.

Other Information Websites

Migraine Awareness Group (MAGNUM)
www.migraines.org

JAMA Migraine Information Center
www.ama-assn.org/special/migraine/migraine.htm

About.com Neuroscience Guide
http//neuroscience.about.com/library/blxDisMig.htm?iam=mt

Migraine Resource Center
www.migrainehelp.com

Headache Impact Test
www.amihealthy.com

Physicians Care Network
www.headachecare.net

Headache Clinic and Information Websites

The New England Center for Headache
www.headachenech.com

The Michigan Headpain and Neurologic Institute
www.mhni.com

The Diamond Headache Clinic
www.diamondheadache.com

Pharmaceutical Company Websites

GlaxoSmithKline (sumatriptan and naratriptan)
www.migrainehelp.com, www.headachetest.com

Merck (rizatriptan, indomethacin, and timolol)
www.maxalt.com

Books on Headache for Patients

The American Council for Headache Education, Constantine LM, Scott S. *Migraine: The Complete Guide*. NY: Dell 2000.

Cady R, Farmer K. *Headache Free*. NY: Bantam Books 1996.

Diamond S, Still B, Still C. *The Hormone Headache*. NY: Macmillan 1995.

Duckro PN, Richardson WD, Marshall JE. *Taking Control of Your Headaches*. NY: The Guilford Press 1995.

Lipton RB, Newman MD, MacLean H. *Migraine: Beating the Odds*. Reading, MA: Addison-Wesley Publishing Company 1992.

Mauskop A, Brill MA. *The Headache Alternative*. NY: Dell 1997.

Rapoport AM, Sheftell FD. *Headache Relief*. NY: Simon and Schuster 1990.

Rapoport AM, Sheftell FD. *Headache Relief for Women*. Boston: Little Brown and Company 1995.

Rapoport AM, Sheftell FD, Tepper SJ. *Conquering Headache*, 4th Edition. Hamilton, Canada: Empowering Press 2002.

Robbins S, Lang SS. *Headache Help*. Boston: Houghton Mifflin 1995.

South V. *Migraine*. Toronto: Key Porter Books 1994.

Index

Page references to figures appear in *italics*.

Understanding Health and Sickness Series
Miriam Bloom, Ph.D., General Editor

Also in this series